THE
HEART
REPAIR
MANUAL

The Philadelphia Formula Program for Preventing and Reversing Atherosclerosis

The Philadelphia Formula

Program for Preventing and

Reversing Atherosclerosis

NICHOLAS L. DE PACE, M.D.

and

STEVEN K. DOWINSKY, M.D.

with Michele Sherman

W·W·NORTON & COMPANY

THE
HEART
REPAIR
MANUAL

NEW YORK · LONDON

Recipes from *Dietitians' Food Favorites* are reprinted with the permission of The American Dietetic Association Foundation. "Refried Beans" and "Bean Enchiladas" from *The 8-Week Cholesterol Cure Cookbook* by Robert Kowalski, copyright (1989) by Robert E. Kowalski. Reprinted by permission of HarperCollins Publishers, Inc. "Black Bean Chili Soup" and "Yogurt Cornbread" from *Weight Watchers Favorite Recipes* by Weight Watchers Int. Inc. Copyright © 1987 by Weight Watchers International, Inc. Used by permission of Dutton Signet, a division of Penguin Books USA Inc.

The text of this book is composed in Melior with the display set in Benguiat Bold.
Composition and manufacturing by the Haddon Craftsmen, Inc.
Book design by Jack Meserole

Library of Congress Cataloging-in-Publication Data
DePace, Nicholas L.
   The heart repair manual : the Philadelphia formula program for preventing and reversing atherosclerosis / by Nicholas L. DePace and Steven K. Dowinsky, with Michele Sherman.
      p. cm.
      1. Coronary heart disease—Prevention. 2. Arteriosclerosis—Prevention. 3. Arteriosclerosis—Diet therapy.
   4. Arteriosclerosis—Exercise therapy. I. Dowinsky, Steven K.
   II. Sherman, Michele. III. Title.
   RC685.C6D452 1993
   616.1′3605—dc20   92-24716

ISBN 0-393-03363-5

W. W. Norton & Company, Inc., 500 Fifth Avenue, New York, N.Y. 10110
W. W. Norton & Company Ltd., 10 Coptic Street, London WC1A 1PU

1 2 3 4 5 6 7 8 9 0

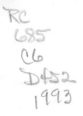

Contents

List of Tables

Authors' Note

Men:

You have opened this book because you're afraid, either because you have atherosclerotic heart disease (hardening of the arteries), or because you fear that what you don't know can kill you. Or, possibly, because your doctor recommended you go on the Philadelphia Formula program. Then again, perhaps your wife, an adult child, or a friend brought the book home, hoping you'd not only read it but use it, wanting you to have your very best chance at staying healthy throughout a long, productive life.

Women:

Your husband may have bought this book for you. It is not only for men. While it's true that, until recently, most of the studies on heart disease were conducted on men, and that most of the literature is aimed at men, women are certainly not immune to coronary (atherosclerotic) heart disease. Of the 550,000 Americans dying each year of heart disease, 250,000 are women. As a result, more and more studies are being conducted on women.

Can we retard and even reverse coronary heart disease? Yes, we can. We do. Read on.

Prologue:
A Worst-Case Scenario

Sam Green's heart stopped beating. An emergency call brought me the news. That's why I was on my way to the hospital in the middle of the night, knowing only too well what I'd probably find when I arrived.

Some months earlier, Sam began having persistent chest pains. His family doctor recommended a cardiologist who, in turn, recommended cardiac catheterization—a procedure during which a film or angiogram of the coronary arteries is made as they are injected with contrast dye. The cardiologist told Sam that the angiogram showed severely blocked coronary arteries. In his opinion, coronary artery bypass surgery was the only treatment offering any hope.

Sam was flabbergasted. He refused to believe it. He decided he needed a second opinion, and remembered his son Evan, a talk radio host, telling him about a cardiologist recently on his program. That cardiologist was me, Nicholas DePace.

Sam set up an appointment and asked me for that second opinion he was convinced would nullify the first. But though he stressed over and over again during the course of my examination that such a terrible thing simply could not be true, his health was excellent, he never even had colds or flu, when I'd finished the examination and reviewed the results of the catheterization, I had to agree bypass surgery was necessary.

Sam's wife Martha, sitting on the edge of a chair beside him in my office, shot a glance at her husband's incredulous face and reached out to squeeze his hand, for her own comfort as much as for his. After forty-five years of marriage, she clearly knew exactly what he was about to say, for she quickly begged him to listen to me and do whatever was necessary.

And so Sam—until the last minute reiterating how well he'd always felt—was operated on by a first-class surgeon. And to everyone's horror, almost every conceivable complication then proceeded to develop. Pneumonia set in, and breathing problems required the prolonged use of a mechanical respirator. Bleeding occurred in the gastrointestinal tract. The surgical wound became infected. The infection spread to the breastbone, which had to be removed, leaving a gaping opening through which the beating heart became visible. More operations were performed in an attempt to repair the chest wall, but Sam was critically ill, his care an ongoing nightmare for both family and physicians.

Now Sam's heart had stopped beating.

There was practically no traffic. It was 3:00 A.M. To be close to Sam, I'd stayed over in my apartment on the top floor of the South Philadelphia Cardiovascular Institute (CVI). Yet the short drive to the hospital seemed to take forever. I tried to distract myself by thinking about medicine's traditional approaches to coronary atherosclerosis—bypass surgery and angioplasty (which uses a balloon catheter to open blocked arteries). Neither of these methods is a panacea. There had to be a better way, and my associate Steven Dowinsky and I believed we finally had the answer.

If only we'd known early on that Sam's arteries were beginning to show serious blockages, he might have been able to avoid bypass surgery. If only we'd had time to start him in the comprehensive atherosclerosis reversal program we would soon be teaching to our first orientation class . . . If only.

Believe me, I knew such thoughts were unproductive and, besides, the hospital was finally in sight. I told myself it was possible I was being unduly pessimistic . . .

In the Coronary Care Unit I ripped off my jacket. Attempts were still being made to resuscitate Sam. I joined the effort, which lasted at least another thirty minutes. Thirty minutes while Sam Green's odds got shorter and shorter, then disappeared.

Finally, there was no choice but to admit it was time to stop trying to revive him. Where there had been frantic activity only moments before while even a tiny hope still existed, now there was the silence of finality. We all stood, drained, looking everywhere except at one another.

I straightened and took a breath. The only thing left to do for Sam was to tell Martha and her children that the struggle had ended.

The Philadelphia Formula
Program for Preventing and
Reversing Atherosclerosis

THE
HEART
REPAIR
MANUAL

Introduction

Philadelphia's revolutionary history isn't limited to politics. The city has also been in the forefront of medical progress with the founding of the nation's first medical college for women, children's hospital, and school of pharmacy. Today, it still boasts some of the country's top medical research and training centers.

One of these is Pennsylvania Hospital, where I've been on staff for many years. The nation's first hospital, it manages to combine the grace and proportion of Federalist architecture with high-tech cardiac facilities ready for the twenty-first century.

It was there in the shadow of its founder, Benjamin Franklin, while I was working on a critically ill patient (long before Sam Green), that I came to the conclusion that America needed a declaration of independence from coronary heart disease— still the number one killer in the country. I wanted to create a program that would get back to basics, taking advantage of our can-do, do-it-yourself spirit. I was convinced that coronary heart disease was not only stoppable but also reversible. A revolutionary idea? Yes. Crazy speculation? Not a bit.

But inspiration is one thing. Taking inspiration that leap further to execution is something else again. The transition demanded intense study of the exact causes of coronary heart disease and heart attacks. I'd pondered these problems while attending the New Jersey School of Medicine, and Mount Sinai Medical School in New York, for my medical degree, and afterward at Hahnemann Medical College and Hospital, in Philadelphia, the site of my residency in internal medicine, as well as a cardiology fellowship. Throughout those years of study I kept telling myself that once the causes (risk factors) of coronary disease were definitely identified, the rest would be easy. All I'd need to ascertain was whether modifying them was within my power as a physician, and if such modification would in any way affect the actual disease process.

On my desk sits a plastic model of the human heart. There have been times when I've sat glaring at it in frustration, trying to order my thoughts. The major risk factors for heart disease have, indeed, become well known fairly recently. So where was the revolutionary program I was supposed to be formulating for my patients and the rest of the world?

I've picked up my little heart and turned it over and over in my hands, knowing the answer was so close. Then I'd get practical and use it with my next patient to help him (or her) visualize how the heart works. I'd explain how the fist-sized heart muscle demands a steady flow of blood to keep up its pumping action. This blood is delivered along a network of small conduits—*coronary arteries.** Like household plumbing pipes, the openings of these arteries can become narrowed—not by rust but by fatty deposits (mainly cholesterol) called *plaque.* This condition is *atherosclerosis* (hardening of the arteries). Should a blood clot *(thrombus)* form at the site of one of these narrowings, a complete blockage results, causing an acute heart attack.

Well, I'm not sure whether one day it was in the middle of such a lecture, or just sitting by myself, but a picture began

*For further discussion of technical terms, see the Glossary (pp. 262–66).

emerging from the tantalizing pieces of this scientific jigsaw puzzle. The picture still wasn't crystal clear, but I was filled with the conviction that coronary heart disease was not a Philadelphia one-way street leading inexorably to heart attacks, bypass surgery, and death. I could make it into a two-way street, offering the hope not only of prevention *but also natural reversal of heart disease,* and I was determined to do just that. You see, I'd begun to view coronary disease as an American epidemic.

Unknown to me, while I was working on my two-way street hypothesis, my future colleague and co-author, Steve Dowinsky, was a continent away in Frankfurt, Germany. He'd received his medical degree from J. W. Goethe University in Frankfurt, and won a research fellowship in cardiology from University Hospital there. All the time I was hoping for a convenient lightbulb to pop on to clear up my confusion over the type of program that would best address my patients' needs, he was analyzing data for the National Institutes of Health. Frankfurt was one of five pioneering centers picked to investigate the effectiveness of coronary angioplasty, a technique which uses a balloon catheter to stretch open narrowed arteries.

Steve's early enthusiasm for this new procedure was soon tempered by the realization that one in four angioplastied narrowings came back within six months. (Cardiologists have since pulled every trick out of their hats to reduce this number, but it's been ten years at least and little has changed.) Coronary bypasses, Steve would learn, were also not immune from becoming diseased and clogged over several years.

The medical profession had to face the fact that the high-tech fixes of bypass surgery and balloon angioplasty were less than permanent. True, this fancy medical plumbing could be life saving, but it in no way changed the disease process that caused the problem in the first place. Our thinking and our management left a lot to be desired.

Steve returned to the United States, and continued his work in coronary atherosclerosis as a clinical fellow in cardiovascular diseases, then started seeing patients. All through this time he was thinking about the need for noninvasive alternatives—a nontechnological strategy to counteract the explosion of bypass surgery and balloon angioplasty. What patients needed was a way to prevent, stabilize, or even reverse the disease process.

When he joined my practice, it proved to be the catalyst we both needed to start developing solutions to the problems. While everyone was jumping on the cholesterol bandwagon, we knew we had to go way beyond controlling total cholesterol to get the results we wanted. Cholesterol was just the tip of the coronary heart disease iceberg.

Knowing that total cholesterol didn't tell the whole story, I developed what we came to call the Philadelphia *Formula.* It's an equation that links together and weights the major modifiable risk factors. It will generate a number—a personalized expression of your relative heart disease risk. This number or score will help your heart whether you're free of heart disease (by driving your score down lower—preventive medicine) or whether you have heart disease (by pushing your score toward zero to help stabilize your sick coronary arteries and even begin to repair them). Our heart repair *program* will give you the tools to beat an unacceptably high score into submission.

If you're telling yourself that a heart repair program like ours is only for sick people, you're dead wrong. Its basic principles are for everyone—young or old, big-bellied or bikinied, whether your blood pressure is high or low, whether your arteries are clogged or wide open.

If you're saying the damage has already been done, I should have started something like this five, ten, maybe twenty years ago, hold on, because we can prove to you that it's never too late. Given half a chance, your heart has the ability to mend itself—something we weren't sure could happen until very recently.

Now I can hear you mumbling that you'll have to give up all

of life's little pleasures to stay healthy. Wrong again! You'll discover that the road to a healthy heart can be paved with enjoyable options. In keeping with Philadelphia tradition, we work hard to preserve your individual freedom of choice. No gurulike dictates from us. We do not expect you to become a strict vegetarian, for example. The good life shouldn't be unpleasantly restrictive nor does it have to be synonymous with an unhealthy lifestyle.

You may be under the impression that the Philadelphia Formula and *Heart Repair Manual* are only for men. After all, much of the early research and reporting on heart disease was traditionally aimed at men. But more than half of the 550,000 Americans dying of heart disease each year are women, and more and more studies are now being conducted on women. Whenever possible, we'll address issues that are specifically related to women and heart disease—like postmenopausal estrogen replacement.

In the years since Sam Green's death, we've applied the Philadelphia Formula heart repair program to many patients, both in individual instruction and group orientation sessions. With the help now of *The Heart Repair Manual,* you, the reader, will eavesdrop on me and Steve as we teach our patients the formula and work out their personalized heart repair programs. We'll take turns guiding you through the chapters, following a representative group of patients (composites of real patients we treat each day), to see how they come to terms with their own risk factors.

You'll soon realize that these risk factors are interlinked. One will create another or make other risk factors worse. The effect is not simply additive. Multiple risk factors multiply the risk of heart disease many-fold. We're going to target those major risk factors that are modifiable—"modifiable" meaning you can do something to change them.

The Major Modifiable Risk Factors

I'm going to list the five major modifiable risk factors by order of the chapters where they appear. This is not their order in the Philadelphia Formula equation, and it does not necessarily connote their relative importance to one another as risk factors for heart disease.

- *High blood pressure (hypertension):* In Chapter 1, we will be discussing your own personalized risk factors, blood pressure, and other topics. Even if your blood pressure is abnormally high, you may not feel anything unusual. That's why hypertension has been dubbed "the silent killer."

    Your heart can tell the difference, though. Lowering your blood pressure, if it is high, is important because high blood pressure stretches and damages the arteries. It also squeezes cholesterol directly into the arterial wall, creating the clogging effect of *plaque.* When forced to pump into a high-pressure system, the heart muscle responds by becoming thicker, a condition called *left ventricular hypertrophy.* This increases your risk of coronary heart disease and sudden cardiac death.

    We want your blood pressure as close to normal as possible (around 120 over 80).

    If you have mild hypertension, we'll offer you non-drug methods to normalize it. For more than mild hypertension, you'll need the help of your doctor to prescribe pressure-lowering medication. We'll guide you through the maze of blood pressure medicines, because some of them can worsen diabetes or even raise your bad cholesterol levels.
- *Total cholesterol:* In Chapters 2 and 3, Steve will discuss cholesterol in the wider context of diet. Your total cholesterol is a number you probably know by now, given the

public's cholesterol awareness. While no one will deny that your risk of heart disease drops with your total cholesterol level, that still doesn't give you the whole picture. If you think that an under-200 total cholesterol level automatically gives you a clean-blood-fat bill of health, you may be sadly mistaken. This is because your total cholesterol reflects not only your "bad" LDL cholesterol level but also your "good" HDL cholesterol, which means that even if your total cholesterol number is under a desirable 200, low levels of "good" HDL put you at significant risk for heart disease.

You have two cholesterol goals on our program. The first will be to drive your "bad" LDL down to about 100, because an LDL this low is effective in reversing atherosclerosis. While heredity plays an important role here, lowering LDL can achieve an overall heart disease risk reduction of just over 20 percent.

Your second cholesterol goal on our program is to bring your "good" HDL cholesterol up to at least 50, because HDL protects against heart disease. There have been a wealth of studies to prove this point. The mammoth Framingham Heart Study, for example, found that low HDL levels were better predictors of heart disease than high total cholesterol levels. And a recent report in the *American Journal of Cardiology* stated that 60 percent of the patients studied with proven coronary disease and total cholesterols under 200 had HDL levels under 35.

Our heart repair program will arm you with HDL-boosting techniques to bring your level to a cardioprotective 50. (People who inherit very high HDL levels—even when total cholesterol is also high—tend to live a very long time.)

Our approach to supercharging your HDL? Regular exercise, weight loss (especially among the big-bellied rather than the fat-fannied), cigarette smoking cessation and passive smoking avoidance (smoke lowers HDL levels), Vitamin C supplements (180 mg a day can bump up levels by 5–10 percent), and for some, modest alcohol consumption.

For others, drugs may be indicated. Estrogen replacement in postmenopausal women with low HDLs can result in increases up to 20 percent. Several cholesterol medications which lower "bad" LDL can also raise "good" HDL (as Steve will show you in Chapter 7).

We'll outline our two-level Nutrition Plan (also in Chapters 2 and 3). The plan should normally effect a reduction in total and LDL cholesterol. But if neither level of the plan gets you to your goal, we'll help you and your doctor choose the best cholesterol-lowering medication.

We'll explain the benefits of heart-smart substances from olive oil and Omega-III fish oil to fiber. You'll learn to become an expert label reader and smart food shopper. Once you know how much fat you should be eating and how much you actually are eating, you won't be duped into eating "hidden" fats.

The Nutrition Plan will make it easier to maintain your ideal body weight without the roller-coaster phenomenon. We'll show you how to figure out what that ideal body weight should be according to the size of your frame. Studies show that a normal body weight reduces the risk of heart attack by 35–55 percent when compared with the body weight of those who are obese (more than 20 percent over ideal body weight).

Obesity and diabetes often go hand in hand. Weight loss and sugar avoidance will help achieve normal blood glucose levels in diabetics. In general, though, you should work with your doctor on these strategies. He or she will decide if sugar-controlling medication is necessary.

• *Exercise:* In Chapter 4, I'll be explaining to you why exercise is a key to weight loss, helping you burn off calories even after you stop working out. Apart from increases in flexibility, strength, coordination, and endurance, a regular exercise regimen has proven to decrease the risk of a heart attack by up to 45 percent. *The Heart Repair Manual* will offer exercise options, even for nonathletes.

You'll learn why we recommend low- to moderate-intensity aerobic exercise. We'll give you an exercise prescription, telling you how often you should work out to get the best results. We'll provide tips on how to prevent exercise-related injuries by following proper warm-up and cool-down techniques.

If you're over forty, we want you to have your doctor perform an exercise stress test before you start any serious workouts. An abnormal test won't necessarily exclude you from exercising, but it may prompt your doctor to recommend additional cardiac studies.

• *Stress:* In Chapter 5, we will discuss stress reduction (which, incidentally, is helped by exercise, for exercise puts our bodies in gear). You must lower your level of stress because stress makes the heart pound faster and harder, raising blood pressure. Job-related stress has been linked by some investigators to hardening of the arteries. Stress-induced surges in the natural stimulant adrenaline can make the heart electrically unstable and cause sudden death. And cholesterol levels tend to rise with stress.

We'll show you how to manage stress through stress reduction techniques such as relaxation therapy.

• *Smoking:* If you're a smoker, the more you smoke, the more you're at risk for heart disease. In Chapter 6, Steve will discuss why you may be finding it hard to quit smoking and why you *must* quit. Quitting smoking is vital, for of the 550,000 people who die of coronary disease every year, 30 to 40 percent can probably blame cigarette smoking. If you smoke, your chances of dying of coronary disease are twice as high as that of nonsmokers.

By the way, women aren't immune. Smoking is probably responsible for nearly half of all heart attacks in women under fifty-five. Smoking directly damages the lining of the coronary arteries and causes blood to clot more easily. Acute heart attacks are usually associated with coronary thrombosis—the formation of a blood clot (thrombus) in a coronary artery.

Quitting smoking is never easy and never quick. Nicotine is powerfully addicting. The Philadelphia Formula offers you a smoking cessation program that's yielded good results with our patients. And be assured—the risk of heart attack drops rapidly once you quit smoking.

Those are the five major modifiable risk factors in the Philadelphia Formula equation. Before we take a look at the equation itself, there's something else we recommend on our program which I want to discuss with you now.

Aspirin

Aspirin has been trumpeted as the miracle drug that keeps on performing miracles, and this is not much of an overstatement for cardiologists. Low-dose aspirin, especially in middle-aged men, reduces the risk of a first heart attack by up to one third. Its blood-thinning effect reduces the chance of clots forming, which helps prevent coronary thrombosis. For those who can tolerate it, aspirin is an integral part of the Philadelphia Formula program.

It's found in most medicine cabinets but, even so, it's not entirely harmless. It can irritate your stomach lining and cause gastrointestinal bleeding, especially in people who have had ulcers. But at the low dosage required to affect blood platelets (a regular adult 325 mg tablet every other day), this won't normally be a factor, and in patients with established atherosclerosis, whose platelets clump together more readily, it is all the more important to take that little aspirin.

Concerning dosage, the Dutch TIA Trial, published in the *New England Journal of Medicine* (October 1991), found that as low a dose as 30 mg of aspirin was equally effective in preventing nonfatal heart attacks, strokes, or death from any vascular source. The study was conducted on selected patients, not a general population of patients with coronary heart disease, and more data is needed before we can recommend this lower dose. However, if you have a history of bleeding problems, specifically gastrointestinal bleeding, you should certainly ask your doctor not only whether you should take aspirin at all, but whether perhaps you might take this very low dose.

Is it really necessary to take an adult 325 mg tablet every other day if you're relatively healthy? The answer is yes for every middle-aged man, even without any history of heart disease, unless major contraindications are present, including allergic reactions like significant rashes or asthmatic attacks, ulcer disease, or bleeding disorder. It should not be taken by patients with hypertension until their blood pressure is brought under control. Your doctor can easily guide you through the potential problem areas.

If you have a strong family history of coronary heart disease or major risk factors such as high cholesterol, cigarette smoking, or diabetes, you should probably be taking aspirin even before middle age. Certainly, you should take aspirin if you're a patient with a history of angina pectoris, heart attack, or bypass surgery.

If you're a woman, the situation is somewhat unclear, for almost all the aspirin studies have included only men. Women are usually at low risk until the onset of menopause at about age fifty to fifty-five. But more information is forthcoming, not only on aspirin but on all aspects of heart disease as it affects women. For example, a study testing aspirin's effectiveness in women began in 1992.

Besides being a blood thinner, aspirin has other beneficial properties that may inhibit atherosclerosis. It has been found to reduce the ability of adrenaline to trigger constriction of the arteries and break down fat, for instance. Also, coronary patients who take aspirin seem to have fewer irregularities in their heart rhythm. And bypasses, when aspirin is used, appear to stay open longer.

Aspirin has been shown to promote the production of interferon, a naturally occurring anti-viral substance, leading some researchers to speculate that if a viral process contributes to atherosclerosis, aspirin may interfere with this mechanism.

Time to Assess Your Own Potential Risk

As you begin reading Chapter 1, and as we figure out your own risk factor score, remember—the risk factors *predispose* you to coronary heart disease. They are not indicators that you already have the disease. I will be showing you the ranges of scores for low, moderate, and high risk, so that you'll know how much work you have to do to become heart-healthy.

Your own doctor will provide you with your cholesterol numbers and blood pressure reading. If you're over forty, he (or she) will have to give you the go-ahead for aerobic exercise. Remember, your doctor, you, Steve, and I are a team. Your primary physician will be glad to provide supervision, when necessary, just as we do for our patients at CVI.

Now that we've run through the basic list of major modifiable risk factors, I'd like to give you a preview of the Philadelphia Formula:

$$\left[\frac{LDL}{10} - \frac{HDL}{5}\right] + 2\left[\frac{\# \text{ OF PACKS}}{\text{PER DAY}}\right] + \frac{\text{EXERCISE}}{\text{SCORE}} + \frac{\text{STRESS}}{\text{SCORE}} + \frac{SBP - 130}{20} = \underline{\hspace{2em}}$$

Don't let the formula put you off. We know that equations have a tendency to bring back memories of high school algebra. But our formula isn't any more difficult than following a cookbook recipe, and it's a lot less scary than figuring out your income taxes. Once you've seen how it's done with the orientation group, you'll realize you don't have to be a math professor to arrive at your Philadelphia Formula score.

Be sure to provide your family doctor with all the information that goes into generating that total number. He/she will want to follow your progress as you begin to move each individual risk factor score toward zero.

Steve and I wrote *The Heart Repair Manual* to equip you with the practical tools you need to start improving your heart's health immediately. Month after month, checkpoint after checkpoint, you'll move closer to your goal of zero cardiac risk. Along the way you'll monitor your blood pressure and cholesterol numbers, painlessly cut your fat and cholesterol intake, stop smoking, exercise aerobically, and manage stress.

Your heart will thank you for doing all this by not developing coronary disease in the first place. More remarkably, though, if you've got any of those artery-narrowing plaques, they can begin to shrink, producing major improvements in blood flow. The scientific evidence is in. The rest is up to you.

1 *Toward Zero*

Locating CVI in South Philadelphia was not whimsical or accidental on my part. South Philly is home to varied ethnic groups. Yet it is nothing if not Italian. It's a place where the old ways still mean something. The residents cling with pride to their little row houses, whose facades echo the skills of artisans with roots reaching back to the old country. The majority of the streets are so narrow, most of them one-way, that only one car at a time can pass.

A fierce sense of community has kept South Philly resistant to the lure of the suburbs, holding the neighborhood and the family intact. All healthy-seeming qualities. So why did I open my cardiovascular clinic in such a neighborhood? My prime reason was the ingrained behavior of a majority of the residents. I hoped through my practice to modify that behavior.

Exactly what behavior do I mean? South Philadelphia (despite its positive qualities) is really a kind of proving ground in terms of the coronary risks its residents subject themselves to. The typical South Philly staples, like fat and cholesterol, smoking, lack of exercise, high blood pressure and stress (sound familiar?), are typical of too many industrialized societies.

Coronary atherosclerosis is a social disease. By that I mean a product of behavior. Fortunately, self-destructive behavior can be controlled. Risk factor intervention can result in prevention.

One week after Sam Green's death, our first orientation class started. The purpose of the group orientation was to instruct several people at once in the Philadelphia Formula heart maintenance and repair program. There were ten members of that first group. (Most groups since have been smaller, so that we can give each member more personal time.) I want you to follow five of the members of the group through the program to illustrate how it actually works.

That first morning, I remember standing over by the wall to greet the class members arriving at the second-floor conference room door. I'd intended this to be a warm room with nothing clinical, businesslike, or threatening about it, so I decided to decorate it with the sort of pictures you probably have scattered around your home—photos, things like that. As the members of that first orientation arrived, it seemed they were pleasantly surprised by the informality of the setting.

I considered what I already knew about these ten people. Five of the men were middle-aged; a sixth was in his thirties and a seventh in his sixties, like Sam. There were also three women: one in her thirties, one postmenopausal, and one elderly. Three members of the group were here because they'd already had a heart attack. But the majority were just scared, for a variety of reasons: because of general health concerns—real or imagined, inconclusive doctors' reports, or conflicting articles on health issues in magazines and newspapers.

I alone would be conducting this session, and many of those to follow. Generally speaking, I see our patients in the office. Steve usually sees them first at the area hospitals.

During this first session, I intended to give a brief outline of the subjects we'd be covering over the next few weeks. Most group members would be able to record small but noticeable improvements in their numbers by the sixth week of following the program; and depending on each one's individual dedication, most should have further substantial improvements in their countdowns toward zero (on which the formula is based) within about nine months.

I knew that the class members, like all of our patients, would find the Nutritional Plan practical, and enjoyable to follow and maintain. The entire program is time-efficient, requiring only an average two hours a week. (This is the total amount of time required for exercise and stress reduction.) The program was created to give all who follow it personalized guidelines on a healthier way to live.

I noticed the youngest woman, Marie Corelli, squirming in her seat. Marie is one of those we will be following through the program. I knew how frightened she was feeling. She had every reason to be frightened. She was here because, two months ago, at the age of only thirty-three, she'd suffered a heart attack. It was Steve who first saw her after that episode while she was still in the hospital. He described that meeting to me.

She was lying there in her bed with two extra blankets over her. The room was warm, but anxiety kept her shivering spasmodically.

"I don't understand." (Because no one ever did.) "I'm young." (Which of course made it that much worse.) "This can't be happening to me. I've always been healthy. I never even had childhood diseases. Everything was good, I was so happy until yesterday. Now, everything's changed."

We hear more or less the same lament over and over. It never gets one iota easier to witness fear like this.

Steve sat down in the visitor's chair beside the bed, holding his clipboard.

"We'll help you change the things that need modification," he told her quietly. "You won't have to do it alone. Some big things, some not so big—daily habits. When you get out of here, we can talk about all that.

"You say you've always been healthy. Nothing you can tell me about? For example, occasional shortness of breath? Pressure or tightness in your chest? Dizziness?"

She hesitated, then, "No. Nothing like that."

He sat back, silent. After a moment, Marie glanced at him, then quickly away. "Just normal things," she mumbled. "Nothing scary."

He left it. His objective wasn't to cross-examine her. But he did ask about the health of her parents.

"Dad's fine. But Mom's been sick a lot for years. I guess nobody took her seriously until she had to have bypass surgery. Oh, and her cholesterol's very high."

So was Marie's. It had already been tested. Steve told her the results, and that it was possible the high cholesterol was hereditary. Toward the end of that first meeting, he suggested cardiac catheterization. He explained that this procedure would show us the condition of her coronary arteries, particularly where the blockages were, how many there were, and how severe they were. He felt it necessary to stress how fortunate she'd been to get to the emergency room in time to be given a clot-busting drug. If the cause of the clot remained unknown, she might not be so lucky next time.

Standing in the conference room, I considered the results of the catheterization. Several of Marie's coronary arteries were severely blocked.

Sam Green's hopeful face superimposed Marie's in my mind—the way he'd looked when I first saw him in my office. I've thought far too often how unfortunate it is that he never had the benefit of the orientation or *The Heart Repair Manual*. But Marie and all the others would. And Marie badly needed major changes in her lifestyle—she was a smoker, ate a cholesterol-rich diet, never exercised. Without these changes she was almost certainly doomed to severe anginal chest pain and repeated heart attacks. The prognosis just wasn't acceptable.

Marie was here for the simplest of reasons. Steve managed

to impress these facts on her and she didn't want to die.

Glancing around the room, I studied all the faces in profile, then went to the front of the room for my opening comments.

"We're unique," I said flatly.

Various murmured conversations stopped and everyone turned toward me.

"How are we unique? Well, first of all, there's nothing bizarre about this program. For example, you're not required to go on a vegetarian diet most of you would probably not want or be able to maintain.

"The entire program's meant to be carried out in the privacy of your own home. This is possible because not everyone needs to follow it to the same degree. In fact, we specifically formulated it so that it can be tailored to your needs, Marie, or yours, Ed—each of you individually.

"We have cholesterol-lowering goals, exercise and stress reduction goals, and if you're a smoker, a smoking cessation program. If you have high blood pressure, we'll work on that, too. When you fill in your risk factor scores, each of you will begin to see clearly which of these factors needs your immediate attention. Some of you may need to start with cholesterol lowering through diet or, possibly, diet plus medication. Others might begin with an exercise program, stress reduction, or stopping smoking. Still others may want to incorporate the whole program into their lifestyle as quickly as possible."

Several of the group members were looking around at each other. One or two were whispering again, their heads close together. I picked up on one of their comments and repeated it out loud.

"So how does that make the formula unique?" I said.

Two of the men glanced at each other, embarrassed. I grinned.

"The Philadelphia Formula is comprehensive, practical, and easy to implement *because it isn't rigid.* If you've ever tried another program like this, you'll realize how unique that is.

Our flexibility lies in the many alternatives available for attaining each goal, as well as in your own ability to judge which goals should be worked on first. There's no group agenda. There's only your own personal agenda, tailored to each of your own needs without requiring radical and unrealistic changes in daily living.

"Also, our program's based on an actual formula—the Philadelphia Formula . . ." I gestured to the equation on the chalkboard behind me

$$\left[\frac{LDL}{10} - \frac{HDL}{5}\right] + 2\left[\begin{matrix}\text{\# OF PACKS}\\\text{PER DAY}\end{matrix}\right] + \text{EXERCISE SCORE} + \text{STRESS SCORE} + \frac{SBP - 130}{20} = \underline{\quad}$$

" . . . with a nine-month timetable for achieving definable end points. By the end of this session, you'll all have filled in your own risk factor scores. Your total score for the five risk factors will tell you whether you're at low, moderate, or high risk for heart disease, and I'll explain that to each of you individually when you complete your calculations.

"By the way, as you'll see, a major factor in the formula is your HDL, your good cholesterol. Most other programs simply mention HDL in a general discussion on cholesterol, with the emphasis on lowering your bad cholesterol, your LDL. In our program, you're forced to follow your good cholesterol as closely as the bad cholesterol. Both are an integral part of the equation.

"The purpose of the program—the formula—is both to reverse hardening of the arteries and to prevent blocked arteries from ever developing in the first place. It's based on the results of many studies carried out all over the world.

"Furthermore, you won't feel you're following this program in a meaningless void. We know that's a problem with so many other programs, having to take it on faith that they're doing you any good. Well, with the Philadelphia Formula, you follow your own progress; no surprises, no mysteries. You'll be noting down how you're doing at regular intervals, starting at six weeks, so you'll be able to watch your risk diminishing at each six-week period *if you're seriously following the program.* You'll do that without needing fancy equipment or a computer or a college degree. And let me assure you, you don't need to be a math whiz or even know much math at all to calculate your scores.

"And finally, if all that's not enough, our program is unique because, unlike so many other programs, the Philadelphia Formula isn't afraid to make promises. These promises require only that you meet quantifiable end points. If all the components of the formula are taken together, you should see significant improvement in your blood chemistry and exercise tolerance within nine weeks. Within nine months the beneficial effects may already be translated into decreased plaque formation and reversal of the existing plaque in your coronary arteries."

I was watching all the members of the group as I spoke. Of the ten, only Ed Donaldson seemed bored and inattentive. He is the second of those I want you to accompany through the program. He was fifty-five, overweight, sedentary, a heavy smoker with high blood pressure, and he'd made it uncomfortably clear he was only there because his wife had nagged him into having a stress test—the test was positive, and then she'd nagged him into joining the orientation. The outlook for such patients usually isn't promising, for they rarely make the effort necessary to modify their habits. There are always a hundred excuses, a thousand procrastinations.

The third class member whose progress we'll watch is Tony Spagnola. He'd suffered chest pains and was under enormous stress at work. The result had finally been a heart attack. Tony was only thirty-two years old.

The fourth member is Carla Peters. She was obese when the class started, a diabetic, and needed not only to lose weight but to lower her LDL, raise her HDL, and start exercising. Six months before the orientation, she'd had a balloon angioplasty of a blocked coronary artery. (This is that procedure during which a balloon is inflated inside the blood vessel to flatten any plaque obstructing and narrowing it.)

And finally, the fifth is Frank Kelsey. Frank was fifty-seven at the time of the orientation. He was happily married, a computer programmer, and he had a secret that was breaking his heart. His reason for joining the group was his high blood pressure. In addition, he had chest pains whenever he exerted himself. He was very unhappy about his problems, desperate to improve.

(As you will see throughout these pages, we will follow not only the scores but some of the impressions our patients have expressed on the program.)

But to get back to that all-important first session, which would hopefully set the tone for the rest of the participants' lives. The next part of the presentation was a brief explanation of the structure and function of the heart. I had my little model with me and now I picked it up. No matter how many times I go through the same talk, I feel it will always be necessary to try to come to it fresh, to keep consciously reaffirming our goals for our patients because, unfortunately, Sam's case wasn't a rare occurrence. Oh, the complications weren't ordinary, but coronary heart disease is frighteningly common. Every year it takes its toll in approximately 1.5 million heart attacks and 550,000 sudden deaths. All the more shocking is that these numbers are not for the whole world, but only for the United States. Approximately 7 million Americans, in that moment I started to speak, had symptomatic heart disease, and 13 million more were walking around as yet undiagnosed.

THE HEART

"The heart pumps over two thousand gallons of blood every day," I began. "Its rate increases with stress or exercise and decreases during sleep. Although considered a single organ, it really consists of two pumps in parallel: the right heart and the left heart. They are joined by a common piece of muscle called the septum.

"The right side of the heart receives blood that is oxygen-poor and contains waste products. It forwards this blood to the lungs, where the oxygen concentration increases from about 70 to 98 percent, and where it is cleaned of carbon dioxide waste. It is then delivered to the left heart.

"The left heart, or left ventricle, is the real workhorse, pumping against very high pressures and resistances to drive the blood through capillaries that may be only $\frac{1}{2,000}$ of an inch in width.

"Over the course of an average lifetime, the heart will pump over one hundred million gallons of blood through the body, a remarkable feat. Because of the amount of work it carries out, the heart muscle requires a constant supply of nutrition in the form of oxygen and other substances, including glucose. These substances are delivered by means of blood transported through the coronary arteries.

"Just after the large artery called the aorta leaves the left heart, it gives rise to two major blood vessels, the left and right coronary arteries, which double back and hug the surface of the heart muscle, resembling the roots of a plant. The coronary arteries have a main trunk and branches, giving off smaller and smaller shoots which eventually tunnel into the heart muscle wall.

"These arteries are usually only a few millimeters in diameter—the size of a small drinking straw. This is why they can become blocked and limit blood flow to the heart muscle. Imagine that you are looking through a drinking straw, through its

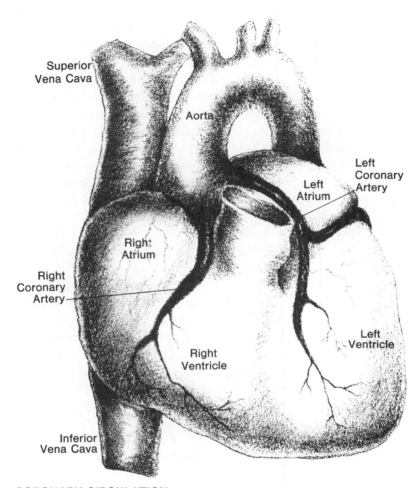

CORONARY CIRCULATION

opening or lumen, and you can easily visualize the caliber of a coronary artery.

"Because the heart is always contracting, the coronary arteries are constantly moving. This puts repeated stress on them and, over time, can cause degenerative changes. Some of this wear and tear is a normal part of the aging process."

I paused for a moment to make sure everyone was following me. There were no questions. I continued.

"Now, imagine that the heart is like an internal combustion engine, and equate the coronary arteries with the fuel line. Any clogging of the fuel line will block the flow of gasoline to the motor, causing it to lose power. The same applies to the heart, which loses efficiency when the coronary arteries cannot deliver blood-borne nutrients. Now you see why a few straw-sized sections of flexible tubing can make the difference between life and death.

"The innermost part of the blood vessel wall consists of cells known as the endothelium protected by a lining called the intima. This inner lining can be damaged by a range of factors from high blood pressure to surgical manipulation.

"Picture the intima as a mesh of fine interwoven shingles. The integrity of this inner lining is vitally important, for it is a kind of protective shield to prevent foreign invaders from penetrating the arterial wall and triggering the atherosclerotic process.

"Coronary artery blockages almost always result from atherosclerosis—an abnormal thickening and hardening within the arteries as a result of the formation of plaques or cobblestonelike deposits called atheromas inside the blood vessel's lining.

"The purpose of the Philadelphia Formula program is to prevent these blockages from ever occurring or, if they are already present, to keep them from progressing. And more—to effect actual regression—reversal, so that the arteries begin to clear, and the flow of blood to the heart continues uninterrupted."

BLOOD PRESSURE

After a few questions and answers, I talked to the class about high blood pressure. Now, I need to discuss it more thoroughly with you than I did in the Introduction.

A lot of our patients with high blood pressure have a hundred silly excuses for not doing anything to correct it. For some of them, medication has proved difficult. This was the case for one of the members of that first orientation: Frank Kelsey. He had a very bad reaction to practically all blood pressure medication.

But it's not true for the majority of people. If you have high blood pressure, you must not ignore your condition, because ignoring it can kill you. Aggressive treatment is necessary. I'm not advocating the quick fix of simply taking a medication and doing nothing else. You need to work on your weight, diet (including your salt intake), lack of exercise, and smoking. All these aspects of the Philadelphia Formula program must be tried, even when medication has been prescribed to lower your blood pressure numbers.

What exactly is blood pressure? It's the pressure exerted by the blood on the wall of any vessel. *Systolic* pressure (the first and higher of the two numbers your doctor records) is the pressure at the height of the pulse wave. It rises during activity or excitement and falls during sleep. Normal in a relaxed, sitting adult is around 120. Your *diastolic* pressure (the second, lower number) is the lowest point to which your pressure drops between beats. Normal is around 80.

It is estimated that 35 million Americans have definite hypertension and 25 million more have borderline hypertension, which makes high blood pressure an enormous health concern in this country. Hypertension runs hand in hand with atherosclerosis and doctors still can't identify any specific cause for this problem in nine out of ten patients. (When this is true, we call it primary or essential hypertension.) It usually becomes evident between the ages of 30 and 50 and it must not be left untreated. Pressures higher than 140/90 mm Hg should be considered for treatment. Over the past twenty years, the number of people whose hypertension has been brought under control has risen from 10 to 50 percent.

The risk of coronary disease rises as blood pressure rises. When blood pressure is high, death from cardiovascular disease is two to three times more frequent than at normal levels. Because of the close relationship of hypertension to coronary heart disease, the outcome of successful treatment of high blood pressure can be stabilization or reversal of coronary heart disease. Reduction of high blood pressure definitely prolongs life. Treating high blood pressure reduces hypertension-related complications such as stroke, heart failure, kidney disease, aneurysms of the aorta, and severe or malignant high blood pressure.

There is no question that one cause of hypertension is the reaction of the sympathetic nervous system to our environment—in other words, stress. However, there are other causes of high blood pressure that are independent of the stress factor. For example, there are genetic factors predisposing some of us to high blood pressure, such as hormone abnormalities (hormones are important in the onset of hypertension). Kidney disease can also cause hypertension, but these are not widespread causes. *For the majority of cases, the cause remains unknown.*

The Philadelphia Formula program deals with your systolic blood pressure number (the one on top), but this does not intimate that the bottom number is unimportant. By treating blood pressure in general, the goal is to normalize both numbers. In fact, it is estimated that a 5–6 point drop in diastolic pressure (the bottom number) reduces heart attacks by 14–17 percent. (But your doctor must monitor this closely, because an excessive drop in diastolic pressure causes an increase in cardiac events.)

Your doctor will also want to keep a close eye on your

reactions to your medication. Some blood pressure medication can increase cholesterol and triglyceride concentrations and reduce high-density lipoprotein cholesterol (HDL) in some patients. For example, drugs such as beta blockers and diuretics can have this effect.

Calcium channel blockers are blood pressure medicines commonly used today. (Calcium acts in contracting the smooth muscle in your blood vessels and therefore can raise your blood pressure.) Calcium channel blockers such as nifedipine, diltiazem, and verapamil obstruct the passage of calcium across the cell membrane. These drugs have also been shown to somehow directly inhibit early atherosclerotic changes. And they decrease the amount of calcium in the cell by cutting down on the constriction of the blood vessel which can cause high blood pressure.

Angiotension-converting inhibitors are also excellent drugs to lower blood pressure. To neutralize some of the bad hormones that can raise blood pressure in your body, drugs such as captopril and enalapril have been used.

If you have high blood pressure, your risk in not taking your medicine is far greater than any minimal side effects you may experience.

Be aware that certain drugs can actually elevate your blood pressure, such as amphetamines, some diet-related products like over-the-counter appetite suppressants, cold and allergy medications (decongestants), and some antacids which contain a lot of sodium. Cortisone products and other types of steroids may also cause a rise in blood pressure, as well as medicines for depression, such as monoamine oxidase inhibitors. The use of oral contraceptives is associated with an elevation in blood pressure in some women. And alcohol consumption can cause blood pressure to rise over short periods.

You must keep in touch with your doctor. This is true whether you have high blood pressure, high cholesterol, experience pain while exercising, are feeling stressed, are a heavy smoker, or have any of a number of other health-related problems needing the attention of a specialist. Your doctor must be informed of your changing health needs, even if you feel they are minor, like taking over-the-counter cold medicines. Once you get into the habit of doing this, it will become second nature; part of that long-term partnership between you and your physician, and in a shorter-term sense, between your doctor, you, Steve, and myself. Such cooperation and communication does not mean losing control over your own life. It means taking control over what happens to you.

End of lecture for the time being. This seems like a good moment to remind you that if you haven't yet done so, you need to go to your family doctor and ask him or her to do a lipoprotein analysis, and to take your blood pressure and tell you your numbers. Also, if necessary, to arrange for an exercise stress test. With this information, we will be able to calculate your Philadelphia Formula risk factor score, as our orientation group members are about to do.

THE PHILADELPHIA FORMULA

The Philadelphia Formula incorporates your scores for cholesterol, smoking, exercise, stress, and blood pressure. Your total score is not a flat judgment condemning you to coronary heart disease, only a baseline value number to follow in our intervention program. In general, a total score of 0 to 4 puts you at low risk; 5 to 10 = moderate risk; above 10 = a high risk of developing or already having coronary heart disease.

Here's the formula, again. So far, we have just talked about it and glanced at it together. Now, I'll explain how to actually use it for your own better health. You'll find your own risk factor sheets at the back of this book, one set to use now for your starting numbers, and six more sets (four pages to each set) for the updates I want you to do for us every six weeks when you see your doctor for a new lipoprotein analysis. Your doctor, you, Steve, and I are partners in this venture, and to assure our success we're going to keep up a constant dialogue.

The risk factor sheets are exactly like those each orientation class member uses to calculate his or her score.

The Philadelphia Formula:

$$\left[\frac{LDL}{10} - \frac{HDL}{5}\right] + 2\left[\begin{array}{c}\text{\# OF PACKS}\\\text{PER DAY}\end{array}\right] + \begin{array}{c}\text{EXERCISE}\\\text{SCORE}\end{array} + \begin{array}{c}\text{STRESS}\\\text{SCORE}\end{array} + \frac{SBP - 130}{20} = \underline{\quad}$$

Now, it's time for me to show you how easy filling in the formula equation really is. Let me explain it to you, step by step. It's very simple. Let's use, for an example, a hypothetical patient, Jeff Alcott. Pictured in purely clinical terms, Jeff looks like this:

Patient Name: Jeff A.
Sex: male
Age: 47
Marital Status: married
Occupation: Administrator, Health Maintenance Organization
Modifiable Risk Factors: Cholesterol—LDL 200; HDL 40
Smoker? Yes. Number of packs/day—2
Activity level—sedentary
Stress level—1⅔
Systolic blood pressure—150

What does all this mean in terms of the Philadelphia Formula equation, and what does it specifically mean to you so that you can use the program? Let's look at that equation again:

$$\left[\frac{LDL}{10} - \frac{HDL}{5}\right] + 2\left[\begin{array}{c}\text{\# OF PACKS}\\\text{PER DAY}\end{array}\right] + \begin{array}{c}\text{EXERCISE}\\\text{SCORE}\end{array} + \begin{array}{c}\text{STRESS}\\\text{SCORE}\end{array} + \frac{SBP - 130}{20} = \underline{\quad}$$

Cholesterol is noted first in the equation. LDL, as we've already explained, is low-density lipoprotein cholesterol. It's the bad cholesterol that's deposited in the artery wall.

HDL is the good, high-density lipoprotein cholesterol. It transports fats out of the liver.

All you really need to know for the purposes of the formula is that you want your LDL as *low* as 100 and your HDL as *high* as possible—we're aiming for at least 50.

Your family doctor has given you the numbers for your LDL and HDL. Enter them now into the equation, on the first set of sheets for your starting numbers. (Remember, all the update sheets are to be found at the back of the book.) Here are Jeff's calculations as an example of how to enter your own numbers:

His LDL is 200. He must divide it by 10 before entering it into the equation. Divided by 10, he gets 20.

His HDL is 40. He must divide it by 5. That gives him an 8 for his HDL.

His LDL minus his HDL would then be 20 − 8 = 12. Those are Jeff's cholesterol numbers. Let's see how they look in the equation:

$$\left[\frac{LDL}{10} - \frac{HDL}{5}\right] + 2\left[\begin{array}{c}\text{\# OF PACKS}\\\text{PER DAY}\end{array}\right] + \begin{array}{c}\text{EXERCISE}\\\text{SCORE}\end{array} + \begin{array}{c}\text{STRESS}\\\text{SCORE}\end{array} + \frac{SBP - 130}{20} = \underline{\quad}$$

$$\left[\frac{200}{10} - \frac{40}{5}\right] + 2\left[\begin{array}{c}\text{\# OF PACKS}\\\text{PER DAY}\end{array}\right] + \begin{array}{c}\text{EXERCISE}\\\text{SCORE}\end{array} + \begin{array}{c}\text{STRESS}\\\text{SCORE}\end{array} + \frac{SBP - 130}{20} = \underline{\quad}$$

$$[\ 20\ -\ 8\ ] + 2\left[\begin{array}{c}\text{\# OF PACKS}\\\text{PER DAY}\end{array}\right] + \begin{array}{c}\text{EXERCISE}\\\text{SCORE}\end{array} + \begin{array}{c}\text{STRESS}\\\text{SCORE}\end{array} + \frac{SBP - 130}{20} = \underline{\quad}$$

The next part of the equation has to do with smoking. If you don't smoke, congratulations! Your score for that is already zero. Jeff smokes two packs a day. He must multiply 2 packs a day by 2. He has a score of 4 for smoking.

$$\left[\frac{LDL}{10} - \frac{HDL}{5}\right] + 2\left[\begin{array}{c}\#\,OF\,PACKS\\PER\,DAY\end{array}\right] + \begin{array}{c}EXERCISE\\SCORE\end{array} + \begin{array}{c}STRESS\\SCORE\end{array} + \frac{SBP - 130}{20} = \underline{\quad}$$

$$[\ 20\ -\ 8\ ] + \quad 4 \quad + \begin{array}{c}EXERCISE\\SCORE\end{array} + \begin{array}{c}STRESS\\SCORE\end{array} + \frac{SBP - 130}{20} = \underline{\quad}$$

Enter your own number on your risk factor sheet. If you smoke now, you'll want to bring it to zero.

Next, exercise. Look at the exercise score sheet to determine your personal exercise score. The sheet will give you the necessary information on how to score yourself, depending on whether you are inactive (sedentary), mildly active, moderately active, or athletic.

Jeff's a couch potato. His activity level was sedentary, giving him the worst possible score of 3.

$$\left[\frac{LDL}{10} - \frac{HDL}{5}\right] + 2\left[\begin{array}{c}\#\,OF\,PACKS\\PER\,DAY\end{array}\right] + \begin{array}{c}EXERCISE\\SCORE\end{array} + \begin{array}{c}STRESS\\SCORE\end{array} + \frac{SBP - 130}{20} = \underline{\quad}$$

$$[\ 20\ -\ 8\ ] + \quad 4 \quad + \quad 3 \quad + \begin{array}{c}STRESS\\SCORE\end{array} + \frac{SBP - 130}{20} = \underline{\quad}$$

Enter your own starting score for exercise.

After the exercise score, we come to stress. Your stress score will be determined by the number of items you check on the personal stress test. You would have the worst possible score if you need to check all 18 possibilities.

Divide the total number of items you checked by 3. That gives you your score for stress. For example, Jeff checked 5 items, then divided by 3, which equals 1⅔. That's his score for stress.

$$\left[\frac{LDL}{10} - \frac{HDL}{5}\right] + 2\left[\begin{array}{c}\#\text{ OF PACKS}\\ \text{PER DAY}\end{array}\right] + \begin{array}{c}\text{EXERCISE}\\ \text{SCORE}\end{array} + \begin{array}{c}\text{STRESS}\\ \text{SCORE}\end{array} + \frac{SBP - 130}{20} = \underline{\hspace{1cm}}$$

$$[\ 20\ -\ 8\ ] + \quad 4 \quad + \quad 3 \quad + \quad 1⅔ \quad + \frac{SBP - 130}{20} = \underline{\hspace{1cm}}$$

What's your stress risk factor score? Fill it in.

Finally, you need to enter the systolic blood pressure (SBP) score you got from your family doctor. Remember, the systolic pressure is the first, higher number. For example, if your blood pressure is 120 over 80, 120 is your systolic pressure.

Now—are you looking at the equation? Write down your systolic pressure on your risk factor sheet, then subtract 130. Jeff has a systolic blood pressure of 150, so his calculation is 150 − 130 = 20. He divides 20 by 20. (Look again at the equation.) His result is 1, so he enters a 1 for his blood pressure score:

$$\left[\frac{LDL}{10} - \frac{HDL}{5}\right] + 2\left[\begin{array}{c}\#\text{ OF PACKS}\\ \text{PER DAY}\end{array}\right] + \begin{array}{c}\text{EXERCISE}\\ \text{SCORE}\end{array} + \begin{array}{c}\text{STRESS}\\ \text{SCORE}\end{array} + \frac{SBP - 130}{20} = \underline{\hspace{1cm}}$$

$$[\ 20\ -\ 8\ ] + \quad 4 \quad + \quad 3 \quad + \quad 1⅔ \quad + \quad 1 \quad = \underline{\hspace{1cm}}$$

Have you filled in your own starting number?

And remember, as you fill in each separate factor score, the higher the number is, the more work you'll have bringing it toward zero. Your end goal is to bring the total of all your scores as close as possible to zero.

Here's how Jeff's numbers added up:

$$\left[\frac{LDL}{10} - \frac{HDL}{5}\right] + 2\left[\frac{\text{\# OF PACKS}}{\text{PER DAY}}\right] + \text{EXERCISE SCORE} + \text{STRESS SCORE} + \frac{SBP - 130}{20} = \underline{\quad}$$

$$[\ 20\ -\ 8\ ] + \quad 4 \quad + \quad 3 \quad + \quad 1\% \quad + \quad 1 \quad = 21\%$$

Because Jeff's total score is very much above 10, he is at high risk. If you've filled in your own numbers you, like Jeff, now know your relative risk and how far you have to go to get to zero.

Are you with me so far? Okay. Then, let's take a look at the orientation group. If you're still confused, the calculations of the five members we're going to follow through the program may help you.

They were all sitting around the conference table filling in their Philadelphia Formula risk scores, just as you're doing. I'd been trying to give Carla Peters a hand. Her attitude concerned me, for it was very negative.

Carla was fifty-three years old at the time of the orientation. She'd been obese all her life, which had resulted in very low self-esteem. Until her angioplasty, she pretty well gave up on ever changing anything.

She had a college background in secondary education, but had taught for only five years before quitting, in favor of positions where she could be less visible and, thereby, feel less vulnerable. At the time she entered our program, she had many health concerns, and was afraid of a multitude of nonhealth-related things as well.

She couldn't concentrate on her risk factor score. She was too focused on worries over what the other members of the group thought of her. She told me her whole life was slipping away, and our program was her last attempt to save herself.

"No one ever sees me for what I am inside, Dr. DePace. All they see is my weight and for some reason they think this entitles them to treat me like a child. This program—it's not for people like me."

"It's for everyone!" Possibly I said it with too much emphasis, for she flinched.

"Everyone," I said, but a good deal more gently, not wishing to frighten her, yet feeling an urgent need to make her care. "It doesn't matter what risk factors you've already accumulated. Of course it's for you. I don't want to hear that."

She shook her head mulishly.

"It's never easy starting new things with new people. We all feel a little nervous," I said truthfully. "But you'll be okay."

She looked up at me.

"You're not alone in this, we're all in it together."

That sounded incredibly trite to my own ears, even though I meant it with all my heart, but she seemed to brighten a little and I left her to fill in her score dubiously. A short time later, she presented me with her risk factor booklet. Here's her calculation:

$$\left[\frac{LDL}{10} - \frac{HDL}{5}\right] + 2\left[\begin{matrix} \# \text{ OF PACKS} \\ \text{PER DAY} \end{matrix}\right] + \begin{matrix} \text{EXERCISE} \\ \text{SCORE} \end{matrix} + \begin{matrix} \text{STRESS} \\ \text{SCORE} \end{matrix} + \frac{SBP - 130}{20} = \underline{\quad}$$

$$[\ 20\ -\ 8\ ] +\qquad 0\qquad +\quad 3\quad +\ 2\ +\qquad 1\qquad = 18$$

I was very pleased to see she didn't smoke, so that was already 0. But unfortunately she didn't exercise either, which gave her the highest possible score of 3. She'd rated herself 2 on her stress analysis, out of a possible 6 (the 18 possible choices divided by 3).

Carla was at high risk for coronary heart disease with her score of 18. She was the first to turn in her material. I looked around to see if anyone else was finished. My attention was drawn to Marie Corelli. She looked terrified. She kept sighing, perhaps hyperventilating, while staring blankly at the papers before her, and her hands were clasped tightly in her lap. I started to go to her to ask if she needed help. But before I could do so, she looked up at me. I smiled and winked, and saw her take a deep, full breath, possibly the first since she'd entered the room. She closed her eyes for a few seconds, and when she opened them again her breathing had slowed almost to normal. She gave me a shaky smile and bent her head over her risk factor booklet.

Here are Marie's starting numbers:

$$\left[\frac{LDL}{10} - \frac{HDL}{5}\right] + 2\left[\begin{array}{c}\text{\# OF PACKS} \\ \text{PER DAY}\end{array}\right] + \text{EXERCISE SCORE} + \text{STRESS SCORE} + \frac{SBP - 130}{20} = \underline{\quad}$$

$$[\ 21 - 8\ ] + \quad 4 \quad + \quad 3 \quad + \quad 2\tfrac{2}{3} \quad + \quad 0 \quad = 22\tfrac{2}{3}$$

Not good, but after all, that was the reason she was here to begin with. Marie was also at high risk.

Tony Spagnola was sitting on the far side of the table from Carla and Marie. Steve and I considered him one of the group members most representative of stress—in his case, occupational stress.

At thirty-two, Tony was the youngest member of the group. He still couldn't believe he'd actually had a heart attack. But he freely admitted that whenever he thought of the job they'd handed him down on his construction site, he got palpitations all over again.

When he gave me his booklet, I saw he'd checked four items on the stress test, for a score of 1⅓. His LDL was already low but, unfortunately, so was his HDL. He had an active job and felt he got enough additional exercise to rate a good low score of 1. But though his total wasn't that bad—just barely above the medium risk category—he sat there staring moodily

at his numbers for some minutes before turning them in, perhaps wondering how his score stacked up to everyone else's:

$$\left[\frac{LDL}{10} - \frac{HDL}{5}\right] + 2\left[\begin{array}{c}\#\text{ OF PACKS}\\ \text{PER DAY}\end{array}\right] + \begin{array}{c}\text{EXERCISE}\\ \text{SCORE}\end{array} + \begin{array}{c}\text{STRESS}\\ \text{SCORE}\end{array} + \frac{SBP - 130}{20} = \underline{\quad}$$

$$[\ 11\ -\ 5\ ] +\quad 2\quad +\quad 1\quad +\ 1\tfrac{1}{3}\ +\quad 0\quad = 10\tfrac{1}{3}$$

Ed Donaldson hadn't looked at his risk factor booklet in a
very long time. When I passed behind him, he looked up and
handed me his finished score. I only realized later that he'd
finished so quickly because he hadn't bothered to calculate it
honestly. He'd just filled in any numbers to get it over and done
with.

His wife Ellen told me a month later that he considered
the program a ridiculous waste of time. She asked me to calculate his real score from the numbers she'd gotten from their
family doctor, which I did. If Ed had taken the trouble to fill
in the real numbers, it would have looked like this (very high
risk):

$$\left[\frac{LDL}{10} - \frac{HDL}{5}\right] + 2\left[\begin{array}{c}\#\text{ OF PACKS}\\ \text{PER DAY}\end{array}\right] + \begin{array}{c}\text{EXERCISE}\\ \text{SCORE}\end{array} + \begin{array}{c}\text{STRESS}\\ \text{SCORE}\end{array} + \frac{SBP - 130}{20} = \underline{\quad}$$

$$[\ 20\ -\ 10\ ] +\quad 6\quad +\quad 3\quad +\ 3\tfrac{2}{3}\ +\quad 2\tfrac{1}{2}\quad = 25\tfrac{1}{6}$$

Frank Kelsey was exhibiting signs of anxiety. He was short
of breath and looked pinched and exhausted. His score was in
the moderately high-risk category:

$$\left[\frac{LDL}{10} - \frac{HDL}{5}\right] + 2\left[\begin{array}{c}\#\text{ OF PACKS}\\ \text{PER DAY}\end{array}\right] + \begin{array}{c}\text{EXERCISE}\\ \text{SCORE}\end{array} + \begin{array}{c}\text{STRESS}\\ \text{SCORE}\end{array} + \frac{SBP - 130}{20} = \underline{\quad}$$

$$[\ 17\ -\ 10\ ] +\quad 0\quad +\quad 3\quad +\quad 1\quad +\quad 3\quad = 14$$

His systolic blood pressure was 190 mm Hg and the medication he'd been taking . . . well, he was mortified by his reaction to his medication. He kept glancing uneasily around at his classmates, as if he feared they'd see right through to the core of his feelings, but as far as I could tell, they were all too involved in their own problems. He handed me his score, then laid his head down on the table as unashamedly as a child might have done.

I later told the group toward the end of the session:

"Know the enemy. If you can recognize the risk factors that foster the development of coronary heart disease, you can delay its emergence or even prevent it ever happening.

"Some risk factors can't be controlled, such as age, sex, and family history. That's the bad news. The older you get, the more likely you are to develop coronary heart disease. Men have CHD more often than women and at younger ages, but women close the gap after menopause. In fact, coronary heart disease ranks first and stroke third as causes of death for women.

"One in seven women aged forty-five to sixty-four have some form of heart disease, and this escalates to one in three over the age of sixty-five. About 10.4 million women of all ages suffer from heart disease and 1.4 million have hardening of the arteries. More than 25 million have high blood pressure.

"Man or woman—If your parents, brothers, or sisters have coronary heart disease before age fifty-five, there's a greater likelihood you'll be affected.

"The good news? You're not locked into your genes. Tendencies may be inherited, but *the major risk factors are modifiable—you can do something to prevent and control them*, by making the decision to alter those daily habits that threaten the health of your heart.

"Up until now, we've only mentioned the major modifiable risk factors we deal with in our equation. But there are others that are relatively less dangerous. A more complete list of modifiable risk factors includes those we've been discussing as well as diabetes and obesity. And although excessive alcohol and caffeine consumption are not considered independent risk factors, cutting down your intake may favorably affect the others.

"Risk factors are cumulative. A universally respected, long-term research project on heart disease, the Framingham Study [see Suggested Readings and Selected References], showed that a forty-year-old man with high blood pressure increased his risk of developing coronary heart disease twofold. Add a very high cholesterol level, and the risk rises tenfold. Throw in mild diabetes, and the risk escalates to twenty-fourfold."

YOUR GOALS

Recognize the characteristics of the enemy. That's your first step. The second is to deal with each separate risk factor as effectively as possible, which means bringing each toward zero. Even modifying a less critical risk factor like obesity is helpful, for losing weight lowers blood pressure, blood sugar, and blood cholesterol. And remember, the goal is not only to stop coronary heart disease in its tracks, but to force its retreat from your coronary arteries.

I'm going to give you some cholesterol goals to strive for as you progress through the program. Remember to use those sheets at the back of this book, not only to enter your starting numbers, but to periodically update your numbers each time you have your cholesterol retested.

You will need to have your cholesterol retested at regular intervals so that you will know whether or not your LDL is coming down and your HDL is rising. I suggest that you have the lipoprotein analysis done every six weeks so that you know what decisions to make at each of these cholesterol checkpoints.

Checkpoint 1 (Six Weeks into the Program)

Begin following the Basic Heart Maintenance phase of the Nutrition Plan, which Steve will detail in Chapters 2 and 3. After six weeks of this level, have your cholesterol test redone. When you get the results, if your LDL hasn't gone down at all, start the Advanced Heart Repair phase. If your LDL number is lower than it was six weeks ago, but not low enough to reach the target of LDL = 100, continue the Basic Heart Maintenance diet for another six weeks. You should be exercising, watching your diet (which means trying to achieve your ideal weight), and if you're a smoker, trying to quit, but it's probably too soon for any of these modifications to have raised a low HDL.

Checkpoint 2 (Twelve Weeks into the Program)

At the twelve-week (three-month) point for your eating plan, have your cholesterol tested again. Is your LDL score moving closer to 100? If your LDL level now = 100 and you accomplished this on the Advanced Heart Repair diet, we want you to simply continue on that level of the Nutrition Plan. If your LDL level is still greater than 100, we want you to add 10 grams of psyllium every day to the Advanced Heart Repair diet, and we want you to have your lipids measured again after another six weeks. It's still too early for noticeable gains in your HDL.

Checkpoint 3 (Eighteen Weeks into the Program)

You've reached four and a half months on the program. If your LDL level is 100 now, continue on the Advanced Heart Repair diet of the eating plan. If you needed psyllium to achieve this goal, continue this level plus the psyllium. If you have not yet reached the LDL goal of 100, your doctor should start drug therapy. In Chapter 7, on cholesterol medication, Steve will explain the cholesterol-reducing drugs. They are primarily for lowering LDL, but several also are beneficial in raising the good HDL. You may be seeing a rise at this time in your HDL, especially if you are following all aspects of the program faithfully. But if your current level of aerobic exercise has had little effect on pushing your HDL closer to 50, try exercising more vigorously, which will also help push the exercise risk factor closer to zero.

Checkpoint 4 (Twenty-four Weeks into the Program)

Six months into the program. If you have already been put on cholesterol medication to try to drive down your LDL level, your cholesterol blood test will tell you whether the medication is working. If it isn't working sufficiently, talk to your doctor about increasing the dose. If your LDL has been lowered by the drug and is now around 100, simply continue your diet plan and the current dose of the drug you are taking. Continue trying to raise your HDL through exercise, and ideal weight maintenance.

Checkpoint 5 (Thirty Weeks into the Program)

Seven and a half months. If your LDL is at the goal of 100, simply continue your diet and drug therapy. If your LDL is still not 100, ask your doctor about adding a second drug to the first. You will want to continue the two-drug combination for another six weeks. How's your HDL? If it's still not moving closer to 50, ask your doctor to consider Niacin therapy. We will be discussing Niacin in Chapter 7 as a drug to both lower LDL and raise HDL. And continue your vigorous exercise program. You should be closing in on zero for that risk factor at this point in the program.

Checkpoint 6 (Thirty-six Weeks into the Program)

You've made it to nine months on the program. It's time for your last official lipid check-in with us. If your LDL is 100, continue your diet and drug therapy. But if your LDL is still not 100, ask your doctor about increasing the dose of the second drug. If even this fails to produce cholesterol levels that will promote reversal of coronary heart disease, your doctor may consider a third drug or an alternative drug therapy.

But no matter what, don't give up. If you stick to the new lifestyle you've fashioned for yourself, your LDL cholesterol will ultimately come down. Regular aerobic exercise, stopping smoking, reduction in stress, and blood pressure control will all combine with your improved eating habits to give you a vastly improved quality of life.

Refer back to these checkpoints when you get to Chapter 3 and start examining the recipes for the Basic Heart Maintenance and Advanced Heart Repair diets. The checkpoints are your guides, so that you will always know when it is necessary to go on to the stricter diet.

Your success in each facet of the program will depend, in great part, on how committed you are to following it. That's the major factor over which Steve and I admittedly have no control: your degree of self-motivation in moving toward zero.

2 *From Shopping Cart to Healthy Heart*

When I joined Nick at CVI it immediately became obvious that to residents and visitors alike, South Philly means food—Italian food and lots of it, from the elegantly burnished woodwork of the four-star Saloon on Seventh Street to Geno's bleached white cheese steak stand. My own favorites aren't the more famous restaurants, but the intimate little trattoria types, often seating less than ten patrons, tucked haphazardly on street corners.

Eating is a competitive sport for South Philadelphians. The trouble is, they often eat the way the Mets play baseball. In a word, badly. The general lifestyle for which this area is known—excessive eating and smoking combined with lack of exercise—keeps the trattorias full. Unfortunately, business at the two neighborhood hospitals straddling South Broad Street is also booming. Booming with a steady stream of heart attack victims. The connection between the dining room and the emergency room, as it turns out, is no coincidence.

South Philadelphia is known throughout the city, and beyond, for a landmark famous for nearly one hundred years— the Italian Market. Here, along Ninth Street, peddlers exhibit their products at curbside before hundreds of small stores selling vegetables and produce, meat, cheeses, and all types of food products—a veritable cornucopia.

Ninth Street starts humming at five in the morning, and the activity goes on until sunset. Throughout the day, trailer trucks, garbage trucks, and all types of freight trucks rumble up and down the street, unloading and picking up merchandise. They are largely ignored by the glut of buyers bargaining with merchants. The majority of these people are not thinking about healthy diets, but they should be.

I cannot stress too strongly that our way of life often determines our way of death. This is especially true of atherosclerosis—the biological rusting out of the heart's plumbing system. But instead of just winding up with a backed-up sink, what we find is obstruction of the coronary arteries—the small pipes which supply the heart muscle with blood. Such clogging causes heart attacks. And heart attacks remain the number one cause of death in South Philadelphia, and for that matter the rest of the country as well.

All this is leading up to our discussion of the Philadelphia Formula Nutrition Plan. Most people eat according to the pleasure principle. But the satisfaction derived from eating is not without risk. Reckless eating, like reckless driving, can be unsafe. The key is to make eating both responsible and pleasurable. That's why we've been so careful not only to define what is most healthy for you to eat, but to provide enough sample recipes to give you the general idea how to create your own unlimited recipes and menus.

We are also well aware that no nutritional plan has a chance of succeeding if it is so difficult to follow that it's not worth the trouble. There are quite a few tables presented in this chapter and in Appendix A (the Fat and Cholesterol Comparison Food Composites). But they're only references—a helping hand as you start to shop and eat more wisely for the health of your heart.

What they must not be is an impediment and a chore. So,

please, remember: Glance at them when you need a reminder, like the amount of saturated fat in a serving of roast beef, or potatoes. Or which fish are highest in Omega-III, or your saturated fat allowance, or your ideal weight.

But never let the tables intimidate you.

By the way, I conducted the orientation class session on nutrition and gave this same pep talk to the group. It turned out to be a very long session, discussing the Nutrition Plan's huge role in pushing that cholesterol risk factor score toward zero. Our eating plan has two levels. Both promote reversal of heart disease by reducing saturated fat and bad LDL cholesterol. You begin with the Basic Heart Maintenance diet, and when necessary, guided by the checkpoints in Chapter 1, progress to the stricter Advanced Heart Repair diet.

I started the session off with two questions:

Do you know whether or not your eating habits are healthy? And what is your diet like now?

If, by any chance, you're still resisting starting the diet phase of the program, how about taking a little quiz to help you assess the fat and cholesterol content of your current diet? Answer the following questions and assign yourself point values for each item (see the key). Remember, this is for you—for your health and long life.

PHILADELPHIA FORMULA SELF-ASSESSMENT QUIZ

KEY: Answer (a) = 1 point (best score)
         Answer (b) = 2 points
         Answer (c) = 3 points

1. What type of fats or oils do you use in cooking?
   (a) I don't use fat or oils in cooking.
   (b) I use margarine and/or vegetable oils in cooking.
   (c) I use butter or butter products, shortening, or lard.

---

2. How often do you eat fried foods?
   (a) I never eat fried foods.
   (b) I eat fried foods once a week.
   (c) I eat fried foods two or more times a week.
3. Cheese consumption per week
   (a) I eat no cheese.
   (b) I use low-fat cheese such as ricotta, low-fat mozza-rella, or low-fat cottage cheese.
   (c) I eat whole milk cheeses such as cheddar, American, or Swiss cheese at least once a week.
4. Type of milk used
   (a) I use only skim or 1% milk.
   (b) I use only 2% milk.
   (c) I use whole milk.
5. Seafood use
   (a) I eat 2 or more servings of fish a week.
   (b) I eat 1 serving of fish a week.
   (c) I rarely eat fish products.
6. Type of spread used on bread, crackers, etc.
   (a) I use soft-tub margarine.
   (b) I use stick margarine.
   (c) I use butter.
7. Number of ounces of meat, fish, or poultry eaten per day
   (a) I do not eat meat, fish, or poultry.
   (b) I eat 4 ounces or less of meat, fish, or poultry per day.
   (c) I eat more than 4 ounces of meat, fish, or poultry per day.
8. Egg yolks
   (a) I avoid egg yolks or use only egg substitutes.
   (b) I eat less than 3 eggs a week.
   (c) I eat more than 3 eggs a week.

9. Snack foods
   (a) I completely avoid snack foods such as potato chips, nuts, crackers, or french fries.
   (b) I eat 1 serving of snack foods a week.
   (c) I eat 2 or more servings of snack foods a week.
10. Baked goods and ice cream
   (a) I completely avoid commercial baked goods and ice cream.
   (b) I eat commercial baked goods or ice cream once a week.
   (c) I eat commercial baked goods or ice cream more than once a week.
11. Fruits and vegetables
   (a) I eat more than 3 servings a day.
   (b) I eat between 1 and 3 servings a day.
   (c) I do not eat fruit or vegetables daily.
12. Consumption of meat products such as beef, pork, lamb, and veal
   (a) I always eat lean cuts or rarely eat meat.
   (b) I occasionally eat lean cuts of meat, but also occasionally eat high-fat cuts, such as hamburgers, spare ribs, sausage, hot dogs, bacon, corned beef, liver, and forms of lunch meat.
   (c) I often eat high-fat cuts of meat.
13. Consumption of split peas, lentils, dried beans, etc.
   (a) I eat these products at least once a week.
   (b) I rarely eat these products.
   (c) I never eat these products.

How did you do? This is one of those occasions when the low man wins. The higher your score, the higher the fat and cholesterol content of your diet. A score of 25 points or less means you're already eating no more than about 300 mg of cholesterol and no more than 30 percent fat, the Basic Heart Maintenance diet.

Let's take a look at the ways in which cholesterol, the bad fats, and salt can negatively affect your heart.

Cholesterol

Dietary cholesterol comes only from animal sources. The classic high-cholesterol foods are whole milk, butter, cheese, egg yolks, liver, brain, kidney, and fatty red meats.

I don't want to give you the impression that cholesterol is a total villain, because it's not. Then what exactly is it? It's a clear, waxy, odorless substance that plays an indispensable role in forming cell membranes and sex hormones. In the form of bile acids, it helps us to digest our food. It insulates nerves and brain tissue. It even makes our skin almost waterproof.

Bad cholesterol (LDL), as you already know, is the type that's deposited right into the coronary artery wall. It's the Mr. Hyde counterpart to the Dr. Jeckyll of good cholesterol (HDL). HDL is the nemesis of LDL, protecting against it much like an environmental crew coping with an oil spill. HDL sucks up surplus cholesterol from blood and tissue cells—even from plaque.

The cholesterol in your blood is either *domestic* (manufactured naturally by your body's cells) or *imported* (dietary). Imported cholesterol comes from eating foods containing saturated fat or pure cholesterol. Most of us can't blame our bodies for producing too much domestic cholesterol. Normally, we produce only what's needed, and the amount is relatively small. For blood vessels, any "trade imbalance" involving excess cholesterol has a detrimental effect. Overloaded with imported cholesterol, arteries begin to become atherosclerotic and clog up.

This is a disturbing picture. How can this rising tide of

cholesterol be stemmed? Obviously, you cannot change your genes if your high cholesterol is hereditary. But the fact that coronary heart disease is rare in underdeveloped countries where the intake of saturated fat and cholesterol is low suggests that our rich Western diet is the primary villain, overwhelming the arterial system to the point of producing disease.

If your high cholesterol is not inherited, you can lower it through diet. If it is hereditary, drugs may be needed. Although women tend to have lower cholesterol levels than men in early life, there's a catch-up phenomenon. Between the ages of forty-five and seventy-four, a total cholesterol count of over 240 creates twice the risk of developing coronary heart disease as a level below 200.

The Bad Fats

Saturated fat, until very recently, received far less publicity than cholesterol. This did not mean it was less dangerous. The term refers to that group of bad fats originating from animal products such as butter, lard, and other animal fats. They're used by the liver to make cholesterol and they are *really* bad for your heart.

Not all vegetable oils are acceptable, either. Some vegetable oils—palm oil, palm kernel oil, and coconut oil (the so-called tropical oils) are loaded with saturated fat.

Nor are all margarines equally healthy. The words "hydrogenated" or "partially hydrogenated" appear on a lot of package listings of ingredients. This refers to margarine or shortening that has been converted from a liquid to a solid. Hydrogenation starts with good unsaturated fat, but the process partly transforms what was good into harmful saturated fat.

Triglycerides

Triglycerides are the major type of fat in the diet. Several different types of studies have determined that a very high level is an independent risk factor for coronary heart disease. Recent data from the Framingham Study indicate that elevated triglycerides constitute a risk for coronary heart disease. For women, such risk is independent of other coronary risk factors. In addition, a Swedish study has also shown that triglyceride levels are an independent risk factor for heart disease.

Other studies refute this finding, making the topic of triglycerides-as-risk factor an area needing further scrutiny before any absolute can be stated.

However, we do know that there are certain disorders of high triglyceride values which do predispose patients to a higher concentration of plaque-forming, small, dense LDL-type particles. In those with such disorders, there is a much higher risk for the development of coronary heart disease.

Also, there is an inverse relationship between triglycerides and HDL. If your triglycerides are high, your HDL tends to be low.

Salt

We're a nation of salt lovers. We must be, considering our dependence on prepackaged, prepared meals and our long-standing devotion to fast food (both of which are, for the most part, loaded with excess salt). And while our bodies need some salt to function properly, what is needed is a fraction of what most of us consume.

Too much salt can cause high blood pressure (hypertension). This is a potentially deadly result of covering our food with layers of whiteness. The average American consumes approximately 4 to 5 grams of salt daily. Three to 4 grams or less is the recommended limit; those with high blood pressure should consume no more than 2 grams daily.

Less deadly, but certainly unpleasant, is the degree to which excessive use of salt can swell body tissues (edema), resulting in a puffy, bloated feeling due to water weight gain, since your body stores this water to try to dilute all that salt. Just think, simply limiting your salt intake can bring about a quick loss of two to five pounds if the weight gain was indeed being caused by water retention.

There is evidence as well that too much salt makes premenstrual tension that much worse, since the symptoms arise largely from the same basic salt plus water retention combination.

I will be discussing the use of salt in your recipes and at the table more fully in Chapter 3.

Now the Good Stuff—The Good Fats

Unsaturated fats are either mono-unsaturated or polyunsaturated, and are found in vegetables or seafood. When you can't get away from eating fat at all, choose items containing these.

Polyunsaturated fats are found in corn, sunflower, safflower, soybean, and cottonseed oils; mono-unsaturated fats in peanut oil, olive oil, and canola (rapeseed) oil. They do not raise cholesterol. Table 1 compares the most often used dietary fats in terms of cholesterol and fat composition.

Another good fat, Omega-III, is found in fish, seafood, and in some plants. A growing number of studies show that eating fish (especially cold-water fish containing the greatest amount of Omega-III fish oil—Table 2) protects against coronary heart disease. It does this in several different ways.

Omega-III consists of long chains of polyunsaturated fatty acids, which enter the food chain when marine algae are eaten by these fish. It has a blood-thinning capability that decreases the possibility of clots forming on plaque. It decreases fibrino-

Table 1
Comparison of Dietary Fats

Fats & Oils (1 tablespoon)	Sat.	Mono.	Poly.	Chol. (mg/tbs)
Olive oil (M)	1.8	9.9	1.1	0
Peanut oil (M)	2.3	6.2	4.3	0
Rapeseed (Canola) (M)	0.9	7.6	4.5	0
Safflower oil (P)	1.2	1.6	10.1	0
Sunflower oil (P)	1.4	2.7	8.9	0
Corn oil (P)	1.7	3.3	8.0	0
Soybean oil (P)	2.0	3.2	7.9	0
Palm oil (S)	6.7	5.0	1.3	0
Palm kernel oil (S)	11.1	1.5	0.2	0
Coconut oil (S)	11.8	0.8	0.2	0
Vegetable shortening (S)	3.2	5.7	3.3	0
Lard (S)	5.0	5.8	1.4	12
Butter (S)	7.1	3.3	0.4	31

M = predominantly mono-unsaturated; P = polyunsaturated; S = saturated
SOURCE: Adapted from *Composition of Foods: Fats and Oils—Raw. Processed. Prepared. Agriculture Handbook* 8-4. U.S. Department of Agriculture, Science and Education Administration (June 1979).

gen levels and can also increase your natural level of tissue plasminogen activator (TPA), a substance produced by the body (and also given as a drug) to *dissolve* a clot once it has formed in the coronary artery. And Omega-III makes red blood cells more flexible, decreasing the stickiness and thickness of the blood.

Omega-III is also available in capsule form but should be taken only under a doctor's supervision. I will explain why, shortly.

Take a look now at Table 2, and also at Table 13 (p. 195) for a comparison of saturated fat and cholesterol in various types of seafood. Make all types of fish, except certain shellfish, a regular part of your diet. Eating moderate amounts of fish has been shown to reduce the rate of coronary heart disease. Try to eat 7 grams a week.

A healthy diet can both lower your bad LDL and raise your good HDL levels—a major goal of the Philadelphia Formula program. Always keep in mind that this dual attack is vitally important. An HDL level below 35 mg/dl puts you at a far greater risk of heart disease than an HDL of 65 mg/dl.

HDL cholesterol can be elevated by dietary means: soluble

Table 2
Omega-III Fatty Acid Composition of Various Fish*

Low (0.5 grams and under)	Medium (0.6 to 1.0 grams)	High (more than 1.0 grams)
Sole	Channel catfish	Rainbow trout
Northern pike	Red snapper	Cisco
Pacific cod	Yellowfish tuna	Pacific mackeral
Atlantic cod	Turbot	Atlantic herring
Walleye	Thread herring	Pacific herring
Yellow perch	Chum salmon	Sardine
Haddock	Striped bass	American eel
Yellowtail	Wolf fish	Sablefish
Sturgeon	Spot	Atlantic salmon
Rockfish	Swordfish	Lake trout
Brook trout	Bluefish	Anchovy
Silver hake	Halibut	Coho salmon
Striped mullet		Pink salmon
Atlantic pollock		Bluefin tuna
Ocean perch		Atlantic mackerel
Carp		King salmon
Weakfish		Spiny dogfish
Skipjack tuna		Albacore tuna
Flounder		Sockeye salmon

*Grams of Omega-III per 100 grams (3½ ounces) of fish, based on data obtained from the U.S. Department of Agriculture.
SOURCE: Adapted from G. L. Becker, *Heart Smart: A Plan for Low-Cholesterol Living* (New York: Simon & Schuster, 1985).

fiber intake, mono-unsaturated fats like olive oil, weight loss, and moderate alcohol intake.

Since We Mentioned Alcohol

Picture a U-shaped curve. Along this curve are three different possibilities, dependent on how much you drink every day. A number of studies show that those who do not drink at all, or who drink only minimal amounts of alcohol, have a slightly higher incidence of coronary disease. This is one end of the U, for those at slightly higher risk. Those who drink moderately have a slightly lower incidence of coronary disease. (Moderate alcohol consumption is defined as one to two drinks per day by the National Institute on Alcohol Abuse and Alcoholism.) This is in the center of the U, the seemingly safest place. But those who drink heavily have a far higher incidence of heart disease, putting them at the other end of the U, at greatly increased risk.

In other words, if you don't drink at all, or only drink minimally, or if you drink heavily, you have a greater risk of heart disease than if you drink moderately.

If drinking moderately does, indeed, have beneficial effects on heart disease, the mechanism by which this occurs is not known. Alcohol may increase HDL levels, but it's not yet clear whether such an alcohol-associated rise in HDL actually has a protective effect.

Please, don't consider any of this a go-ahead toward alcoholism. For one thing, too many health problems are related to heavy drinking. Alcohol can raise triglycerides and blood pressure; in excess, it can cause weakening of the heart muscle. In addition, we are all aware of the numerous social problems that can occur when alcohol intake exceeds a certain level. This can add a stress factor which may promote atherosclerosis and be counterproductive.

All the conflicting studies are undeniably confusing. Our position is this: If you are a moderate or light drinker, there is no reason to stop this level of drinking unless you are hypertensive, have high triglycerides, or are significantly overweight and need to avoid the calories. If you are a heavy drinker, you must curtail your intake immediately. If you do not drink or drink only minimally, we do not recommend increasing your alcohol intake. There are better methods for preventing and reversing heart disease than taking a drink a day.

What Do You Know About Dietary Fiber?

There's been a lot in the news recently about dietary fiber and cholesterol. There are two types of dietary fiber: *soluble* and *insoluble.* All foods containing fiber are a mixture of both types. High-fiber foods (complex carbohydrates), which are low in saturated fat, are the best foods you can eat. A glance at Table 3 will give you an idea of the relative amounts of soluble and insoluble fiber in a variety of items. You can see, for example, that oatmeal (rolled oats) is almost 14 percent total fiber, of which 7.7 is soluble fiber. A quick look at the food composite for bread, cereal, etc. (see Table 18, p. 205) gives you the further information that a single cup serving of oatmeal contains 145 calories, no cholesterol, low saturated fat—an excellent choice for breakfast.

What's the difference between soluble and insoluble fiber?

Insoluble fiber (or roughage) represents about 70 percent of the total fiber in a normal diet. It adds bulk to the stool but has little or no cholesterol-lowering effect. However, insoluble fiber has been shown to decrease the risk of colon cancer by speeding up elimination of waste products. It also has a laxative effect that decreases the risk of developing hemorrhoids.

It is low in calories and high in bulk, filling you up quickly and reducing hunger pangs. That makes it a valuable part of any weight reduction program.

Soluble fiber is the type that blocks the uptake of dietary "imported" cholesterol and bile acids from the intestine. This

Table 3

Fiber Content of Various Foods

	% Total Plant Fiber	% Insoluble Fiber	% Soluble Fiber
Wheat bran	42.2	38.9	3.3
Oat bran	27.8	13.8	14.0
Oats (rolled oats)	13.9	6.2	7.7
Corn flakes	12.2	5.0	7.2
Grapenuts	13.0	7.4	5.6
Pinto bean	10.5	6.0	4.5
White bean	7.7	4.0	3.7
Kidney bean	10.2	5.5	4.7
Lima bean	9.7	6.4	3.3
Corn	3.3	1.5	1.8
Sweet potato	2.5	1.4	1.1
Kale	2.6	2.0	0.6
Asparagus	1.6	1.1	0.5
Cucumber	0.9	0.5	0.4
Apple	2.0	1.1	0.9
Orange	2.0	1.4	0.6
Banana	1.8	1.0	0.8
Peach	1.4	1.1	0.3

SOURCE: J. W. Anderson and W. J. Chen, "Plant fiber: Carbohydrate and lipid metabolism." *American Journal of Clinical Nutrition* 32(2):346–63, February 1979.

lowers blood levels of LDL cholesterol and may increase good HDL cholesterol. Soluble fiber is found in fresh fruits and vegetables, whole grain breads and cereals.

You should have 15 to 18 grams of soluble fiber daily. You can supplement your dietary intake with psyllium (products like Metamucil, Fiberall, Konsyl, and some house brands you'll find in your local drug or health food store). They are available over the counter, but remember, they're meant only to be a supplement. Most of your 15–18 grams a day should come from the food you eat, as part of your healthy diet.

By the way, the laxative effect of psyllium helps prevent gas, diarrhea, or constipation—discomforts you may temporarily experience when first changing to a high-fiber diet.

A word about oat bran. Oat bran's real effectiveness in reducing cholesterol has remained controversial. Still, it's been shown to work when cholesterol levels are over 230 mg/dl. Otherwise, oat bran serves as a good substitute for foods containing saturated fat.

To control most cholesterol problems, you really must restrict your dietary cholesterol and saturated fat, use soluble fiber, control your weight, and exercise regularly. These decisions are in your hands. If you try everything, but your cholesterol remains too high, don't give up. You may simply need to talk to your doctor about appropriate medication to help with the problem.

You and Your Ideal Weight

You may be under the impression that if you don't need to lose weight, you can ignore the whole process of watching your saturated fat and cholesterol intake, and of shopping more wisely for your food. But whether you need to diet for weight loss or not, you still need to know the actual number of calories to allow for fat in whatever you're eating every day. And you must be aware of the saturated fat content and cholesterol in everything you eat.

To determine if you need to lose weight, look at Tables 4A and 4B.

To determine whether your frame is small, medium, or large, clasp the thumb and middle finger of your left hand around your right wrist. If they don't meet, you have a large frame. If they just barely touch—medium. If you can easily wrap your fingers around your wrist, your frame is small.

Table 4A

Desirable Weights (Ages 25 and Over): Men*
1983 Metropolitan Height and Weight Tables

Height		Small Frame	Medium Frame	Large Frame
Feet	*Inches*			
5	2	128–134	131–141	138–150
5	3	130–136	133–143	140–153
5	4	132–138	135–145	142–156
5	5	134–140	137–148	144–160
5	6	136–142	139–151	146–164
5	7	138–145	142–154	149–168
5	8	140–148	145–157	152–172
5	9	142–151	148–160	155–176
5	10	144–154	151–163	158–180
5	11	146–157	154–166	161–184
6	0	149–160	157–170	164–188
6	1	152–164	160–174	168–192
6	2	155–168	164–178	172–197
6	3	158–172	167–182	176–202
6	4	162–176	171–187	181–207

*Weight in pounds according to frame (in indoor clothing weighing 5 lbs., shoes with 1″ heels).

SOURCE: 1979 Build Study, Society of Actuaries and Association of Life Insurance Medical Directories of America, 1980.

Now, look at Table 5A or 5B to determine the maximum number of grams of saturated fat you should consume each day for *your ideal weight*. Find the figure in the left-hand column that most closely corresponds to your desirable weight. Then move across the chart to the vertical column that corresponds to your level of physical activity. This is your personal grams of saturated fat (GSF) number. It applies to a 10 percent saturated fat diet (Basic Heart Maintenance diet). The number in parenthesis will apply if you need to progress to the Advanced Heart Repair diet.

Table 4B
Desirable Weights (Ages 25 and Over): Women*
1983 Metropolitan Height and Weight Tables

Height		Small Frame	Medium Frame	Large Frame
Feet	*Inches*			
4	10	102–111	109–121	118–131
4	11	103–113	111–123	120–134
5	0	104–115	113–126	122–137
5	1	106–118	115–129	125–140
5	2	108–121	118–132	128–143
5	3	111–124	121–135	131–147
5	4	114–127	124–138	134–151
5	5	117–130	127–141	137–155
5	6	120–133	130–144	140–159
5	7	123–136	133–147	143–163
5	8	126–139	136–150	146–167
5	9	129–142	139–153	149–170
5	10	132–145	142–156	152–173
5	11	135–148	145–159	155–176
6	0	138–151	148–162	158–179

*Weight in pounds according to frame (in indoor clothing weighing 3 lbs., shoes with 1″ heels).
SOURCE: 1979 Build Study, Society of Actuaries and Association of Life Insurance Medical Directors of America, 1980.

Let me give you an example of how to use Table 4A or 4B in conjunction with Table 5A or 5B.

Let's say you're a sedentary woman (you don't get any exercise), whose height is 5′2″ and whose frame is small. Look at Table 4B.

As you can see, a 5′2″ woman, small-framed, should weigh between 108 and 121 pounds. That's her ideal weight range. Now, look at Table 5A, if you're a man, or Table 5B if you're a woman, for the number of grams of saturated fat you are allowed, depending on your ideal weight and on your level of

Table 5A
GSF Numbers: Men/Activity Level

Desirable Weight	Sedentary	Moderately Active	Sports
90	14 (10)	15 (11)	16 (12)
100	16 (12)	17 (12.5)	18 (13)
110	17 (12.5)	18 (13)	20 (14.5)
120	19 (13.5)	20 (14.5)	21 (15)
130	20 (14.5)	22 (15)	23 (15.5)
140	22 (16)	23 (16.5)	25 (18)
150	23 (16.5)	25 (18)	27 (19)
160	25 (18)	27 (19)	28 (20)
170	26 (18.5)	28 (20)	30 (21)
180	28 (20)	30 (21)	32 (22.5)
190	30 (21)	32 (22.5)	34 (24)
200	31 (22)	33 (23)	36 (25)
210	33 (23)	35 (24.5)	37 (26)
220	34 (24)	37 (26)	38 (26.5)

SOURCE: Modified from Art Ulene, *Count Out Cholesterol: American Medical Association Campaign Against Cholesterol. Feeling Fine* (New York: Random House, 1989).

physical activity. The woman in our example is sedentary. At the upper level of her ideal weight range, 121 pounds, she is allowed no more than 17 grams of saturated fat daily on the Basic Heart Maintenance diet and only 12.5 on the Advanced Heart Repair diet.

Do this simple numbers check for your own height, weight, and activity level.

Obesity as a Minor Risk Factor

If you recall, I mentioned earlier that obesity is one of the minor modifiable risk factors. If you determine from the tables that you do need to diet, whether you need to lose only a few pounds or much more than that, take a look now at Table 6, to

Table 5B
GSF Numbers: Women/Activity Level

Desirable Weight	Sedentary	Moderately Active	Sports
90	13 (9.5)	14 (10.0)	14 (10.0)
100	14 (10.0)	15 (11)	16 (12)
110	15 (11)	17 (12.5)	18 (13)
120	17 (12.5)	18 (13)	19 (13.5)
130	18 (13)	20 (14.5)	21 (15)
140	20 (14.5)	21 (15)	22 (16)
150	21 (15)	23 (16.5)	24 (17)
160	22 (16)	24 (17)	26 (18.5)
170	24 (17)	26 (18.5)	27 (19)
180	25 (18)	27 (19)	29 (20.5)
190	27 (19)	29 (20.5)	30 (21)
200	28 (20)	30 (21)	32 (22.5)
210	29 (20.5)	32 (22.5)	34 (24)
220	31 (22)	33 (23)	35 (24.5)

SOURCE: Modified from Art Ulene, *Count Out Cholesterol: American Medical Association Campaign Against Cholesterol. Feeling Fine.*

determine the number of total grams of fat allowed at the caloric-intake level you will attempt. All this may sound alarming, but believe me, it's not. The tables were designed to make it easy.

Table 6 simply shows you what 30 percent fat (the amount allowed on the Basic Heart Maintenance diet) actually means in grams of fat at different calorie levels. For example, if you are on a 1,200 calorie a day diet, the lowest reasonable number of calories if you're to be successful, you should consume no more than 36 grams of fat, and only one third of that—12 grams—may be saturated fat.

If you need to lose weight, you have plenty of company. Millions of Americans, both men and women, are on that eternal roller coaster, a physical and emotional "upper" (shedding

Table 6
Calories/Grams of Fat

Calories Daily	Grams of Fat (= *30%*)
1200	36
1500	45
1800	54
2000	60
2500	75
3000	90

pounds) and "downer" (gaining them back). This roller coaster ride is, unfortunately, self-perpetuating since dieters rarely make a permanent change in their eating habits, resulting in a return to the old ways as soon as the scale shows an attractive drop in pounds.

My point, of course, is that you need to revamp the entire way you view your normal diet if your hard-won weight loss is to be permanent. A reversal of obesity and a maintenance of weight loss both follow automatically for anyone who undertakes the Philadelphia Formula Nutrition Plan, along with the accompanying recommended aerobic exercise program and stress reduction techniques. But if you have been considering other diets, especially fad diets that typically promise the world in a very short time with little or no discomfort to you, remember this: In order to affect weight loss, a diet must first satisfy the need for energy; second, be tasty; and third, minimize hunger and fatigue.

A Warning About Fad Diets

There are definite dangers in some fad diets. Very low calorie diets (less than 800 calories a day) are often protein-poor. Sudden death has occurred in some cases, presumably brought on by low potassium and cardiac arrhythmias. Besides, losing weight rapidly on diets like this means you'll tend to gain it back with equal rapidity when the diet "ends." This can lower your resting metabolic rate, making it even more difficult to lose weight the next time you attempt it.

Many weight reduction programs fail: only one out of twenty patients manage to maintain a loss of 25 pounds or more after two years. If you're serious about losing weight, and keeping it off, this is hardly an acceptable ratio.

Less than 1,200 calories a day is unreasonable and creates rampant hunger, leading to a tendency to cheat. To be successful, *a diet must be linked to exercise and stress reduction techniques.*

There are several commercial and self-help programs available. Some are properly supervised, others are not. Most don't keep exercise diaries or emphasize aerobic exercise programs, for their concern is solely caloric intake. Many start well below that 1,200 calories a day lower limit, and many are impractical and expensive as well.

Some programs offer prepared foods, so the dieter never learns to deal with reality; others use a protein-sparing program with a powder diet formula. But some protein-sparing diets allow only 400 to 800 calories and do not initially stress exercise. Most are too restrictive, and fail to instill dietary habits that people can maintain out in the real world.

Just be wary of any program promising dramatic weight reduction in a short period of time. If the program doesn't incorporate permanent lifestyle changes, it's almost certain to fail. The use of diuretics, thyroid, or other hormone manipulations, and amino acid supplements should be avoided as well.

Three Patients Respond

Carla presented Nick with a write-up we think you'll find helpful in using some of the tables. He had her on the Basic Heart

Maintenance diet, and in three weeks she'd already lost 10 pounds. She was extremely excited. She'd tried powder diets and special freezer foods before, but on our program, simply limiting her saturated fat (which automatically limited her calories) was leading to her first dieting success.

Her note presented a typical day as the old Carla. This is what she reported:

> On the Basic Heart Maintenance diet, I could eat no more than 20½ grams of saturated fat a day. I found that out by looking at the sheet that lists grams of saturated fat for my desired weight (145 lbs) according to my exercise level, which was sedentary (Table 5B).
>
> I used the food composites listing cholesterol and saturated fat comparisons to calculate what I'd been used to eating. It really grossed me out!
>
> For breakfast I'd been having: two large waffles: 8 grams of saturated fat (Table 18); an 8-ounce glass of whole milk: 5.1 grams (Table 14).
>
> That made it 13 1 grams of saturated fat just for breakfast out of my total for the whole day of 20. Pretty scary, wasn't it?
>
> For lunch I'd been used to eating: two sandwiches of turkey roll on whole wheat bread—that I figure had more than 3½ ounces of turkey roll in each sandwich; but the chart lists what a normal serving should be, so: 2 grams (Table 12). (Two sandwiches, 2 times 2 grams = 4 grams just for the turkey roll.) A slice of bread: 0.4 grams (Table 18). (Four slices = 1.6 grams. That made my lunch 5.6 grams of saturated fat. Breakfast and lunch together—18.7 grams.
>
> Dinner was always another quickie, things I liked that were easy, for example: 2 hot dogs and lots of black coffee. Hot dog buns: 0.5 grams each (Table 18) = 1 gram. Two frankfurters (Table 11) = 12 grams. My easy dinner came to 13 grams.
>
> Totaling up the entire day, what did I have? A whopping 31.7 grams of saturated fat. And while I'm being so honest, I might as well tell you that I didn't include dessert, and I always had dessert. I really love cream pie, and I always took more than ⅓ of the pie,

not the listed ⅙ (Table 19). My dessert alone came to at least 30 grams of saturated fat, making the grand total by bedtime around 61 grams. And I'm not done confessing yet, because in the middle of the night, I'd almost always get up for a snack.

You see, I don't mind telling you all that now, because it's history. Since I've been on the Basic Heart Maintenance diet, I think I've gotten a sort of grip on myself. Now that I know why I'm overweight, why my cholesterol was high, I can do something about it. I know I'll never be three times my saturated fat allowance again, because maybe this doesn't make sense; but the very thought of all that fat swimming around in my blood, clogging up my arteries, makes me sick enough to want to throw up.

I hope Carla's note helps you to realize how easy it is to use the tables if you haven't already found that out for yourself. What makes it easy, I assure you, is that all you need to do is choose as many items from the top of each category on Tables 11–20 as possible. Those are the ones with the least saturated fat. And choose as few from the bottom of the lists as possible, for they are heaviest with saturated fat.

You will have very little dependence on the tables once you've started internalizing the numbers on those items you eat most often. So don't get frustrated, in the beginning, while you're still learning. Frustration can lead to quitting, and the worst thing you can do is give up.

Marie and I had a talk about her early attempts to change her eating habits. Her experience was less positive. Her family, particularly her husband, was not supportive. She said:

"My husband James, said, 'This chicken isn't the way I like it.' You see, I always used to fry everything, and this time I baked the chicken without the skin.

"Anyway, he had an attitude all the time he was eating it. He told me he still expects me to make my deep-fried zucchini and mushrooms, and everything else I used to always cook with tons of eggs and cheese. I told him I'm already learning new recipes, and in my heart I know he really won't be able to tell the difference, not if he's honest, but I'm afraid he won't be.

"I love to eat as much as he does, and I try never to fool myself. Why won't people admit that using low-fat ingredients doesn't change the taste, except for making it, I don't know, somehow cleaner. Do you know what I mean?"

I remember Nick saying that self-motivation was the one thing neither he nor I could control. But there's obviously more than one thing, as you can see from my discussion with Marie. Family support, especially at the start of lifestyle changes, is vitally important. It can make all the difference between success and failure, particularly if the patient is tentative about undertaking the program.

Finally, Frank Kelsey talked to Nick about his new diet, specifically Omega-III fish oils. He gave us his blessing in telling you his secret, for it's no longer a problem for him.

For the past six years, he'd been on one blood pressure medication after another. Every one had side effects. Fatigue was the most insidious; the lethargy was terrible at work, with friends, at home. But the most horrible and shameful to his mind was his impotence on almost all the medications.

Although he'd tried to deny it to himself, the impotence seriously damaged Frank's image of himself as a man. It was the reason he'd joined the CVI program, in the hope that we could somehow cure what nothing else had.

All his family doctor's tests, as well as our own, failed to pinpoint the cause for his hypertension. He had generally elevated blood pressure, cause unknown. All of his earlier attempts to reduce his salt intake, to exercise—he'd been using a stationary bike at home, but had to stop after very little exertion due to chest pains—and to maintain his ideal weight, had had little effect on his blood pressure.

For that reason, Nick started him on fish oil capsules. Now, let me make this clear. Neither Nick nor I like fish oil capsules. I'll explain why in a minute. We would have vastly preferred our usual route of using an anti-hypertensive. In Frank's case, it was his call, because of his past experiences on these medications and the anxiety he felt at the very thought of taking yet another of them.

But Nick did warn him that it was safer and healthier to eat 7 grams of Omega-III fish a week, and that he should seriously try to incorporate such fish into his diet and get off the fish oil capsules as quickly as possible.

At any rate, Frank did start the fish oil capsules, and after only a month of fish oil, the Philadelphia Formula Basic Heart Maintenance diet and the walk program (Table 7), his LDL had already dropped from 170 to 150. And best of all, his blood pressure, which had been 190/110, was now 130/90 with absolutely no side effects.

(Although Frank did see his LDL cholesterol level go down, fish oils generally do not cause significant reductions in LDL. Far more dramatic is their ability to lower triglyceride levels.)

Frank proudly reported his sex life was back to normal, perhaps better than normal after losing it for so long. But what was most telling was that psychologically he felt great, for he was on a near-natural substance. He assured us he was starting to eat Omega-III fish, particularly salmon and tuna. He enjoyed them both, and it could hardly be called a sacrifice to substitute them two or three times a week for beef.

As you know from your earlier reading in this chapter, Omega-III's help in lowering Frank's blood pressure isn't by any means its only benefit, though that alone would be substantial. Fish oils have been found to lower blood pressure both in people with high and with normal blood pressure. Decreasing an elevated blood pressure eliminates a cause of trauma to the blood vessel wall which, if it continued, could damage the endothelium and trigger the atherosclerotic process.

About Fish Oil Capsules

Fish oil capsules are sold over the counter, so they seem perfectly safe, and they *are* if used in the appropriate dosage. But the tendency on the part of lots of people is to take too many of them, in order to avoid eating fish—something I firmly believe is nothing but a remembered childhood aversion.

If you plan to take fish oil capsules, consult your doctor first, especially if you're on additional medication, including aspirin. The capsules can have side effects when taken in large doses. For example, too high a dose might make you susceptible to stroke with bleeding. And if you're a diabetic, fish oils should be avoided, because of their undesirable effects on insulin secretion and glucose production. Large doses can also cause considerable weight gain.

Pesticides such as mercury may have accumulated in the bodies of the fish being used, accumulations which could then be concentrated in the fish oil capsules. Taking large doses of them may be unwise.

There are no real risks in eating fresh, uncontaminated fish, and there are so many delicious and varied dishes that a dieter should have no difficulty finding quite a few new favorites.

3 A Nutritional Survival Guide

Between six and seven in the morning, the small luncheonettes throughout South Philadelphia are crammed with people wolfing down breakfast before going to work. Eggs and bacon, sausage and ham, caffeinated coffee with loads of sugar and cream, rich doughnuts, and everything else that's disastrous for the heart is consumed at these breakfasts. Lunch and dinner, for most of them, are no healthier than breakfast.

Nick and I sometimes grab a quick cup of coffee on our way to CVI or to one or another of the local hospitals. So we find ourselves watching those around us indulge in these suicidal eating habits. There's no excuse for eating like this *besides* habit, because there's a tremendous variety of wonderful food available.

The restaurants, large and small, in South Philly offer the fish catches of the day, pastas with and without heavy cream sauces, the best Italian wines, fantastic bread. What it comes down to is basically this: Two things are necessary before you can eat properly. You have to want to do so, and you have to be aware of what healthy eating means in terms of the choices you make, so that you can move your cholesterol score toward zero.

LABEL-READING

Intelligent food shopping is being made easier than it used to be, nutritionally speaking. For this we can thank all the current concerns over fat and cholesterol. Information on the amount and type of fat, percentage of calories derived from fat, cholesterol, and fiber content now appears on most of the food produced and packaged in the United States.

Some products don't yet have these new labels. But even without them, you can still shop wisely and carefully. With the help of Table 3 (Fiber Content, p. 55) and Appendix A, Tables 11–20 (the Fat and Cholesterol Comparison Charts), you'll be well informed about a vast variety of foods. Again, these tables are your servants, not your masters.

On package labels, the ingredient present in the largest amount, by weight, has to be listed first. It will then be followed in descending order of weight by the other ingredients. As you shop, check out the relative proportions of polyunsaturated, mono-unsaturated, and saturated fat, and choose items with as little saturated fat as possible. If an item lists more than 2 grams of saturated fat per cup or serving, it's best to avoid that product. Total fat should be near the bottom of the list, or better yet, not present at all.

Foods low in saturated fat also tend to be low in dietary cholesterol, but there are exceptions, for example, liver, shrimp, and eggs. You'll see this clearly in Tables 11–20. On both the Basic Heart Maintenance and the Advanced Heart Repair diets there are maximum amounts you should allow for fat and cholesterol. We will discuss this shortly, before taking a look at the menus and recipes in this chapter.

As you shop, keep in mind what's acceptable and what's not on those product ingredient labels. Items to avoid: butter, chocolate, cocoa butter, coconut or coconut butter or coconut oil, cream, egg yolks, saturated fat, hydrogenated fat, lard, palm or palm kernel oil, and shortening. We'd like you to try to avoid these completely, even if they appear at the bottom of the label. If you can't manage that yet, at least eat products containing them sparingly if you're on the Basic Heart Maintenance diet. For the Advanced Heart Repair diet, egg yolks, for example, are not allowed at all, and you would be wise to teach yourself to avoid all the above items entirely.

On the other hand, there are many items it is acceptable to select on product labels. For example: canola (rapeseed) oil, corn oil, olive oil, safflower oil, sesame oil, soybean oil (include partially hydrogenated), sunflower oil, skim milk, nonfat dried milk products, diglycerides, hydrolyzed products, and mono-glycerides.

Replacements for dietary fat (fat replacers) are intended to reduce the fat content in food while still providing the sort of high-fat taste and texture many consumers demand. They are usually carbohydrate, fatty acid, or protein-based, and include polysaccharide carrageenin, which has been used for centuries and can be found in dessert pie fillings, yogurt, and sauces, and is even used now by fast-food chains in low-fat ground beef. They, too, are acceptable.

Avoid foods listing a high sugar content. Choose high-fiber foods—complex carbohydrates. These are often the first foods eliminated by dieters, which is a big mistake, for doing so will only make you tired and sluggish. Complex carbohydrates produce energy. And besides, they're relatively low in calories. A half cup of cooked pasta, a single slice of bread, three-quarters of a cup of dry cereal, or a half cup of mashed potatoes (go very easy on the margarine and skim milk when you prepare them), each contain only about 70 calories. It's the size of the portion that will make or break your diet.

GENERAL SHOPPING GUIDE

Meat, poultry, fish, and shellfish are all excellent sources of vitamins, minerals, and protein. Depending on the type and cut, they contain varying quantities of cholesterol (Tables 12, 13, and 14). Choose only the leanest types of meat. In beef: round, chuck, sirloin, and loin; in veal: all trimmed cuts; in pork: tenderloin, leg, or shoulder; in lamb: arm and loin. Avoid well-marbled cuts of meat with excess fat around the edges, and most organ meats like liver, which are high in cholesterol.

There are different grades of meat. Prime contains the most fat; choice has less marbling. Look for labels that say "lower fat," "lean," "extra lean," or "lite," and make sure they list less than 60 percent of their calories from fat. Avoid all processed meats such as bologna, sausage, hot dogs, salami, and bacon.

Chicken and turkey are low in saturated fat and cholesterol. Remove the skin *before* cooking, for most of the fat is found in the skin. And choose white meat over dark if you want to save calories.

Milk and cheese (Table 14) contain proteins and many vitamins. However, whole milk contains significant amounts of saturated fat and cholesterol. Skim and low-fat milk (1 or 2%) have the same nutritional value as whole milk. When buying cheese, avoid processed and imitation cheeses and cheese spreads. Instead of cream cheese, try Neufchatel cheese. Natural and hard cheeses (like Cheddar) are highest in saturated fat. Try low-fat, part-skim mozzarella and ricotta, and low-fat (1%) cottage cheese and farmer's cheese.

Before you reach for that carton of eggs, be aware that one egg yolk contains approximately 274 mg of cholesterol (Table 14). On the Basic Heart Maintenance diet, you should limit yourself to no more than two eggs a week. No eggs are allowed on the Advanced Heart Repair diet.

Egg whites contain no cholesterol and are high in protein. Egg Beaters consist of 99 percent real egg whites. Try making omelettes using egg substitute, two egg whites, or a combination of both for every whole egg. Chopped boiled egg whites make a good garnish for salads.

Fruits and vegetables are low in fat and calories and contain no cholesterol. Try to buy fresh fruit and fresh or unprepared frozen vegetables rather than canned or commercially prepared frozen vegetables, which contain large amounts of salt as well as hidden fat. Read the labels carefully.

When you're shopping, don't pass up the fresh fish counter (Table 13). All fish, and especially Omega-III-rich fish (Table 2), should be a part of your diet.

Avoid most regular pre-mixed salad dressings; they're high in fat. There are more and more fat-free, cholesterol-free salad dressings for you to sample. Or you might use vinegar and a polyunsaturated oil such as corn oil. Try fat-free, cholesterol-free mayonnaise in your tuna salad.

Bread and cereal products (Tables 3 and 18) like rice— especially brown rice, which is high in soluble fiber—pasta, beans, and peas all contain lots of vitamins and fiber. In breads, the greatest amount of fiber is in the whole grain types. Water bagels are delicious, as well as English muffins, pita bread, unsalted pretzels, crackers, and matzo (not egg matzo).

Be careful to avoid commercially prepared baked goods such as doughnuts, muffins, croissants, biscuits, and butter rolls, which probably contain eggs and large amounts of saturated fat. Other items to avoid: anything made with whole eggs, heavy cream, whole milk, butter, and lard. Potato chips, corn chips, or microwave popcorn with added fat are not recommended.

Ice cream, long an American favorite, is high in calories, saturated fat, and cholesterol (Table 15). Instead, check out frozen yogurt, which has become an extremely popular alternative to ice cream due to its lower calories, lower fat and cholesterol. Frozen yogurt is widely available in the supermarket and yogurt/ice-cream shops (found in malls and shopping centers). Selections include both nonfat and low-fat varieties. For the Advanced Heart Repair diet, only the nonfat frozen yogurt is recommended. Some shops include a nonfat, sugar-free variety sweetened with Nutrasweet if you want additional reduction in calories. You'll only need to sample it once to find that frozen yogurt is a satisfying and delicious snack or dessert with a variety of flavors offered for your selection.

Water ices, popsicles, and fruit sorbets are also good low-fat desserts, as are gelatin and puddings made with skim milk. Air-popped popcorn, angel-food cake, ginger snaps, and vanilla wafers are all good choices. Also, several companies now have no-fat, no-cholesterol, low-calorie cookies and cakes. Or you may want to bake your own, using heart-healthy ingredients.

Be aware, also, of your salt usage. As you will see, very few of our recipes include salt as an ingredient. Instead, we suggest the use of a variety of herbs and spices to keep meals healthy and interesting.

Sodium is listed in milligrams on food labels (1 gram = 1,000 milligrams). Choose food items containing less than 200 mgs per serving. Food labels may also include any of the following terms: "sodium-free" = less than 5 mg per serving; "very low sodium" = 36 mg or less per serving; "low sodium" = 140 mg or less; "reduced sodium" = 75 percent less than in a comparable item; "salt-free" = no salt added during processing.

Avoid foods such as sardines, smoked ham, bacon, and processed luncheon meats, and try to cut back on snacking foods topped with salt such as pretzels, pumpkin seeds, and saltines, and condiments like ketchup, which contains high amounts of salt and should be used only sparingly.

Try low-sodium seasonings. You might make your own "salt shaker" by combining herbs and spices such as pepper, garlic powder, onion powder, oregano, chives, cloves, paprika, tarragon, ginger, curry powder, sage, bay leaf, parsley, rosemary, basil, and thyme.

Now, this is the most important point. When following a low-cholesterol, low-fat, high-fiber, low-salt diet, you *must* be sure to eat a wide variety of foods so that you get all the vitamins, minerals, and nutrients you need to stay healthy. For example, eat oat bran, but don't ignore other fiber sources like rye bread or whole wheat pasta. And remember, red meat shouldn't normally be excluded from your diet. It's high in iron and protein. A balanced diet will help you reach your dietary goals.

If you've followed these guidelines, and Tables 11–20, you've selected healthy food items. But your job's not finished by a long shot. Now, it's time to prepare what you've purchased. Your goal is to choose those methods of food preparation that will keep as low as possible both the level of fat and the number of calories in the finished product you put on your table.

GENERAL COOKING GUIDE

Baking, broiling, grilling, and roasting on a rack are the healthiest ways to cook your meats, poultry, and fish. The rack allows excess fat to drip away from meats and poultry.

Avoid deep frying. Occasionally, you might want to fry your foods lightly in a small amount of polyunsaturated oil, using flour instead of breadcrumbs. (Breadcrumbs tend to absorb more fat.)

Stir-frying (wok) or sautéeing can be done using water instead of oil. You may also consider nonstick vegetable sprays for pan-frying (for example, when you make an omelette using egg substitute and/or egg whites, or if you are preparing boneless, skinless chicken breast). Such nonstick vegetable sprays add only a minimal number of calories and fat.

Try using nonstick pans, as well, for pan-frying without any fat at all. And when you do use oil, make it the polyunsaturated or mono-unsaturated types (Tables 1 and 16). Avoid lard, butter, and solid shortenings. If you use margarine, make it the soft-tub type, because stick margarines become more saturated during the process of hydrogenation.

Trim off excess fat from the edges of your meat and remove the skin from poultry before cooking. To keep chicken moist without the skin, try marinating it overnight in a fat-free salad dressing. While roasting or baking your meats without the skin, try wrapping or covering them with aluminum foil, or occasionally basting with water, fat-free salad dressing, broth, or natural juice gravies. Avoid adding heavy sauces and creams.

Chill soups (both homemade and canned) overnight and skim off the fat that rises to the surface before reheating and serving.

The sample recipes that follow in this chapter provide specific instructions on how best to prepare your food so that it remains healthy.

THE NUTRITION PLANS

These eating plans should be considered permanent, not temporary.

The Basic Heart Maintenance diet limits cholesterol to no more than 300 mg a day, fat to no more than 30 percent of total calories (at ideal weight), and saturated fat to no more than 10 percent of total calories. You are allowed two eggs a week, meat, poultry, and seafood in amounts of approximately 6–7 ounces a day, but you should limit your use of organ meats like liver, and you may use mayonnaise, Thousand Island, and other commercial dressings. Meatless alternatives are not necessary.

The Advanced Heart Repair diet limits cholesterol to no more than 150 mg a day, fat to no more than 23 percent of total calories (at ideal weight), and saturated fat to no more than approximately 7 percent of total calories. No eggs at all are allowed, meatless alternatives are required, servings of meat, poultry, and seafood should be no more than 3–4 ounces a day, you must avoid organ meats completely, as well as mayonnaise and commercial dressings, but you may use canola oil and olive oil in their place. Just a few examples of the many meatless possibilities include cheese (skim milk, low-fat), beans, lentils, and egg substitute.

The checkpoints in Chapter 1, starting on p. 39, tell you when you need to progress from the Basic Heart Maintenance to the Advanced Heart Repair diet. Now, enjoy the sample menus and recipes in the following pages. They will give you an idea of the wide range of possibilities on both the Basic Heart Maintenance and the Advanced Heart Repair diets.

Items with an asterisk indicate that recipes are provided. These were contributed by a number of individuals. Use the fat and cholesterol comparison food composites in Appendix A to be sure of getting as little saturated fat as possible in your diet as you create your own unlimited recipes. Simply choose items closer to the top than to the bottom of each category on each list.

And remember, feel free to be creative. It's always better to use fresh seasonings, such as fresh garlic instead of garlic powder, and fresh homemade items such as your own tomato sauce rather than the jar or canned types, which usually contain a lot of sugar and/or salt. When seasoning your food, be careful of salt, but use fresh herbs and spices to please your own taste.

A gratifying number of cookbooks include low-fat, low-cholesterol recipes, and the number is growing as we all become more aware of the need to prepare and consume healthy food. *The New American Diet,* by S. L. and W. E. Connor; *One Meal at a Time,* by M. Katahn; and *The Don't Eat Your Heart Out Cookbook,* by J. C. Piscatella, are just a few you'll find in your bookstore.

If going through the Nutrition Program fails to lower your cholesterol level enough to make regression possible, drug therapy should be started. This will most often be considered only after at least three months of diet have failed; but when very high LDL cholesterol levels or severe coronary heart disease are evident from the outset, your doctor may wish to add supplemental drug therapy to your diet sooner rather than later. Drug therapy should always be *added* to dietary therapy, not simply substituted for it. I will discuss the various cholesterol medications with you in Chapter 7, if this is what you need to bring your cholesterol score toward zero.

BASIC HEART MAINTENANCE DIET

Sample 1

BREAKFAST
1 glass **Grapefruit Juice**
1 **Egg**, any style
1 **Bagel**
1 teaspoon soft-tub **Margarine**
½ cup **Skim Milk**
Decaffeinated **Coffee** or **Tea**

LUNCH
½ cup **Chicken Broth** with
½ cup of **Pastine**
Chicken Salad (2 oz chicken, 2 tsp
mayonnaise, chopped celery)
Lettuce, Tomato
2 slices **Pumpernickel Bread**
1 **Pear**
3 **Graham Crackers**
Decaffeinated **Coffee** or **Tea**

DINNER
*1 **Italian Manicotti** with tomato sauce
*¾ cup **Zucchini Italienne**
½ cup **Beets**
1 cup **Orange and Grapefruit Sections**
1 cup **Skim Milk**
Decaffeinated **Coffee** or **Tea**

Italian Manicotti with Tomato Sauce

Ingredients	5 Portions	Method
Manicotti shells, 5-inch	5	Cook according to package directions; drain.
Frozen chopped spinach, thawed, drained well	1 10-oz package	Combine. Stuff shells; arrange in baking pan coated with vegetable spray.
Cottage cheese, drained	1 cup	
Egg substitute, = beaten	2 eggs	
Onion, pared, chopped	¼ cup	
Garlic powder	½ cup	
Oregano	1 tsp	
Thyme	⅛ tsp	
Tomato sauce	1 cup	Pour over shells.
Mozzarella cheese, shredded	4 oz	Top with. Cover; bake at 350F for 25 minutes or until done. Serving size: 1 shell.

Italian Manicotti with Tomato Sauce   (Continued)

Nutrient Analysis

Calories	249
Total Fat	8 gr
Fiber	1.4 gr
Cholesterol	116 mg

SOURCE: Members of the American Dietetic Association. *Dietitians' Food Favorites* (Des Plaines, IL: Cahners Publishing Co., 1985).

Zucchini Italienne

Ingredients	3 Portions	Method
Zucchini squash, sliced	2 cups	Combine in skillet. Simmer, covered, 20 minutes or until tender.
Black olives, pitted	¼ cup	
Italian dressing, low calorie	⅛ cup	
Pimento	⅛ cup	Add before serving. Serving size: ¾ cup.

Nutrient Analysis

Calories	40
Total Fat	2.4 gr
Fiber	1.0 gr
Cholesterol	0 mg

SOURCE: Members of the American Dietetic Association. *Dietitians' Food Favorites.*

BASIC HEART MAINTENANCE DIET

Sample 2

BREAKFAST 1 glass **Orange Juice**
1 **Egg,** any style
2 slices **Raisin Bread**
1 teaspoon soft-tub **Margarine**
½ cup **Skim Milk**
Decaffeinated Coffee or **Tea**

LUNCH *1 cup **Tomato Florentine Soup**
6 unsalted **Crackers**
Meatball Sandwich (2 oz lean ground beef,
⅓ cup tomato sauce)
1 **Italian Roll**
Tossed Salad (1 cup raw vegetables)
Fat-Free Dressing
*¼ cup **Pineapple Frappe**

DINNER *½ breast of **Chicken Italiano**
½ cup **Broccoli Rabe**
1 cup **Pasta** (1 tsp olive oil)
½ cup **Pudding** (made with skim milk)
2 **Plums**
½ cup **Skim Milk**
Decaffeinated Coffee or **Tea**

Tomato Florentine Soup

Ingredients	5 Portions	Method
Tomato juice	2 cups	Combine; heat to
Beef broth or	1½ cups	boiling. Reduce heat;
consommé		simmer for about 30
Water	1½ cups	minutes.
Frozen chopped	5 oz	Serving size: 1 cup.
spinach		
Onion, pared, minced	⅛ cup	

Nutrient Analysis

Calories	34
Total Fat	0.2 gr
Fiber	1.0 gr
Cholesterol	7 mg

SOURCE: Members of the American Dietetic Association. *Dietitians' Food Favorites.*

Pineapple Frappe

Ingredients	4 Portions	Method
Pineapple juice, canned, unsweetened	½ cup	Combine all ingredients into blender and blend until smooth. Pour
Pineapple, fresh or canned, drained	2¼ cups	sherbet into a shallow pan and place in freezer.
Buttermilk	1½ tsp	Freeze overnight. Next
Vanilla extract	¼ tsp	day, thaw to a mushy
Lemon juice	½ tsp	consistency and blend
Artificial sweetener	to taste	again to incorporate air and keep ice crystals small. Refreeze until ready to serve. Serve in sherbet glasses. Serving size: ¼ cup.

Nutrient Analysis

Calories	62
Total Fat	0.4 gr
Fiber	1.4 gr
Cholesterol	0 mg

SOURCE: Members of the American Dietetic Association. *Dietitians' Food Favorites.*

Chicken Breast Italiano

Ingredients	3 Portions	Method
Boneless, skinless chicken breasts, cut in half, each half 3–4 oz	1½	Lightly pound until flattened.
Sun-dried tomato halves, packed in olive oil, drained	6	Place 2 tomato halves and 1 artichoke heart on each breast. Roll up; secure with wooden pick. Place in frying pan or casserole.
Marinated artichoke hearts, drained	3	
Chicken stock	1 cup	Pour over; heat, covered, over low heat about 20 minutes until tender. Remove from stock; heat until reduced. Serve chicken sliced across into 4 pieces.
White wine	1 cup	
Fresh parsley, chopped	1 Tbsp	Pour hot broth over; sprinkle with parsley and basil. Serving size: ½ breast.
Fresh basil or oregano, chopped	1½ tsp	

Chicken Breast Italiano   (Continued)

Nutrient Analysis

Calories	362
Total Fat	6.8 gr
Fiber	3.4 gr
Cholesterol	68 mg

SOURCE: Members of the American Dietetic Association. *Dietitians' Food Favorites.*

BASIC HEART MAINTENANCE DIET

Sample 3

BREAKFAST   ½ cup **Cranberry Juice**
1 cup **Melon Balls**
1 **Egg,** any style
½ cup **Rice Krispies**
1 slice **Whole Wheat Bread**
1 teaspoon soft-tub **Margarine**
½ cup **Skim Milk**

LUNCH   *1½ cups **Minestrone Soup**
2 ounces fresh **Turkey,** lettuce, tomato
1 **Pita Pocket**
1 tablespoon fat-free **Mayonnaise**
1 cup **Fruited Gelatin**
2 **Ginger Snaps**
Decaffeinated **Coffee** or **Tea**

DINNER   *8 ounces **Maine Fish Stew**
1 slice **French Bread**
1 teaspoon soft-tub **Margarine**
½ cup steamed **Broccoli**
15 **Grapes**
½ cup nonfat **Frozen Yogurt**
½ cup **Skim Milk**
Decaffeinated **Coffee** or **Tea**

Minestrone Soup

Ingredients	4 Portions	Method
Dry navy beans	¼ cup	Combine in large
Chicken stock	⅔ cup	kettle. Cook for 1
Water	1 pint	hour.
Carrots, pared, cut in strips	2	Add; cook for 30 minutes. Reserve.
Potato, pared, diced	1	
Cabbage, shredded	¼ lb	
Canned tomatoes, low salt	1 8-oz can	
Onion, pared, sliced	½	Sauté until
Olive oil	2½ tsp	translucent.
Celery rib, sliced	½	Add; sauté until
Zucchini, sliced	½ lb	tender. Stir into bean
Garlic clove, pared, mashed	1	mixture.
Pepper	dash	
Basil	¼ tsp	
Marjoram	⅛ tsp	
Parsley, fresh, chopped	1 Tbsp	Add; cook for 20 minutes. Add more
Tomato sauce, low salt	¼ cup	water if too thick.
Spaghetti, broken	¼ cup	Add: cook for 10 minutes. Serving size: 1½ cups.

Minestrone Soup   (Continued)

Nutrient Analysis	
Calories	164
Total Fat	3.4 gr
Fiber	4.9 gr
Cholesterol	0 mg

SOURCE: Members of the American Dietetic Association. *Dietitians' Food Favorites.*

Maine Fish Stew

Ingredients	4 Portions	Method
Medium onion, pared, chopped	1	Sauté in kettle for 5 minutes.
Carrots, pared, cut into ¼" dice	½ cup	
Celery, cut into ¼" dice	½ cup	
Garlic clove, pared, minced	1	
Olive oil	2½ Tbsp	
Potatoes, pared, cut into ½" dice	1½ cups	Add; cook for 5 minutes more.
White wine	1 cup	

Maine Fish Stew (Continued)

Ingredients	4 Portions	Method
Fish stock	1 cup	Add; simmer, covered,
Whole peeled tomatoes	1 cup	for 25 minutes.
Tomato paste	2 Tbsp	
Bay leaf	1	
Thyme	½ tsp	
Tabasco sauce	¼ tsp	
Cod fillets, cut into 1" pieces	1¼ lb	Add; simmer, uncovered, for 10 minutes more.
Parsley, chopped	¼ cup	Top with. Bottled clam juice can be substituted for fish stock. Pollock, haddock, or hake fillets can be substituted for cod. Serving size: 8 oz.

Nutrient Analysis	
Calories	284
Total Fat	9.4 gr
Fiber	1.3 gr
Cholesterol	0 mg

SOURCE: Members of the American Dietetic Association. *Dietitians' Food Favorites.*

BASIC HEART MAINTENANCE DIET

Sample 4

BREAKFAST ⅓ cup **Apricot Nectar**
1 **Egg,** any style
½ cup **Bran Cereal**
½ **Sesame Bagel**
1 teaspoon soft-tub **Margarine**
½ **Banana**
Decaffeinated **Coffee** or **Tea**

LUNCH **Macaroni Tuna Salad** (2 oz water-packed
tuna, ½ cup macaroni, 1 tsp fat-free
mayonnaise)
6 **Breadsticks**
½ cup **Celery Sticks**
½ cup fresh **Fruit Salad**
3 cups plain **Popcorn**
Decaffeinated **Coffee** or **Tea**

DINNER 1 cup **Chicken Noodle Soup**
*4 ounces **Eggplant Strata**
*½ cup **Zucchini-Carrot Julienne**
1 slice **Whole Wheat Bread**
1 teaspoon soft-tub **Margarine**
1¼ cup **Watermelon**
1 cup **Skim Milk**
Decaffeinated **Coffee** or **Tea**

Eggplant Strata

Ingredients	4 Portions	Method
Eggplant, pared, cut lengthwise into ½″ thick slices	1¼ lb	Soak eggplant for 30 minutes in enough lightly salted water to cover. Rinse with cold water; pat dry. Arrange in single layer on nonstick baking sheet; broil about 5 minutes on each side until tender.
Water	As needed	
Salt	To taste	
Green pepper, thinly sliced	½	Sauté lightly in nonstick skillet.
Large onion, pared, thinly sliced	½	
Green beans, fresh cut, blanched	½ lb	Add to sautéed vegetables; combine.
Part-skim ricotta cheese	½ lb	Combine. Arrange half of eggplant slices in baking dishes sprayed with nonstick cooking spray. Cover with vegetable mixture.
Scallions, thinly sliced	¼ cup	
Plain low-fat yogurt	⅛ cup	
Dried oregano leaves, crushed	⅛ tsp	Sprinkle on. Spoon on cheese mixture. Top with remaining eggplant.
Garlic powder	Pinch	

Eggplant Strata (Continued)

Ingredients	4 Portions	Method
Tomato sauce	4 oz	Pour over.
Mozzarella cheese	2 oz	Sprinkle on.
Tomato, thinly sliced	1	Arrange on top.
Parmesan cheese, grated	1 tsp	Sprinkle on. Bake at 350F for 35 minutes until bubbly. Blanched zucchini slices can be added with, or in place of, green beans. One cup of cooked rice can be added as an additional layer. Serving size: 4 oz.

Nutrient Analysis

Calories	214
Total Fat	8.1 gr
Fiber	4.0 gr
Cholesterol	29 mg

SOURCE: Members of the American Dietetic Association. *Dietitians' Food Favorites.*

Zucchini-Carrot Julienne

Ingredients	6 Portions	Method
Large zucchini, cut into julienne strips	1	Steam or cook vegetables in small amount of water for 15 to 20 minutes or until tender.
Large carrots, pared cut into julienne strips	2	
Boiling water	As needed	Drain.
Margarine	2 tsp	Add; toss to coat.
Dill weed	½ tsp	Top with. Serving size: ½ cup.

Nutrient Analysis

Calories	38
Total Fat	1.5 gr
Fiber	1.0 gr
Cholesterol	0 mg

SOURCE: Members of the American Dietetic Association. *Dietitians' Food Favorites.*

BASIC HEART MAINTENANCE DIET

Sample 5

BREAKFAST   ½ cup **Grapefruit Juice**
1 **Egg**, any style
½ cup **Bran Flakes**
1 slice **Whole Grain Bread**
1 teaspoon soft-tub **Margarine**
½ cup **Skim Milk**
Decaffeinated **Coffee** or **Tea**

LUNCH   *¾ cup **Gazpacho Soup**
*1 **Bean Enchilada**
½ cup **Brown Rice**
1 tsp soft-tub **Margarine**
½ cup **Applesauce**
Decaffeinated **Coffee** or **Tea**

DINNER   *3 ounces **Chicken and Rice**
*½ cup **Refried Beans**
½ cup **Carrots**
1 **Roll**
1 teaspoon soft-tub **Margarine**
½ cup **Nonfat Frozen Yogurt**
½ cup **Skim Milk**
15 **Grapes**

Gazpacho Soup

Ingredients	4 Portions	Method
Vegetable cocktail juice	23 oz	Place in blender or food processor;
Wine vinegar	¼ cup	process until blended.
White vinegar	⅛ cup	
Sherry	⅛ cup	
Lemon juice	1 Tbsp	
Olive oil	1 Tbsp	
Worcestershire sauce	½ Tbsp	
Hot pepper sauce	To taste	
Medium cucumber, pared, cut into small cubes	1	Combine thoroughly; stir in liquid. Refrigerate, covered,
Large ripe tomato, cut into cubes	1	for 4 hours. Serve in chilled bowls or
Large green bell pepper, chopped	½	mugs.
Medium onion, pared, chopped	¼	Serving size: ¾ cup.
Prepared onion soup base	¾	
Parsley, chopped	1¼ Tbsp	
Celery salt	⅛ tsp	
Freshly ground white pepper	¼ tsp	
Garlic cloves, crushed	1 tsp	

Gazpacho Soup   (Continued)

Nutrient Analysis

Calories	129
Total Fat	4.5 gr
Fiber	1.8 gr
Cholesterol	0 mg

SOURCE: Members of the American Dietetic Association. *Dietitians' Food Favorites.*

Bean Enchiladas

Ingredients	6 Portions	Method
Onion, chopped	½ cup	Sauté until softened in large skillet, using nonstick spray.
Chicken breast, cut into ½" squares	8 oz	Combine. Simmer until chicken is
Black beans, drained	1-lb can	cooked. Cool.
Green chilies, chopped	4 oz	

Bean Enchiladas (Continued)

Ingredients	6 Portions	Method
Cilantro or parsley, fresh, chopped	½ cup	Add to mixture.
Corn tortillas	12	Heat gently. Spoon filling mixture along one edge of each and roll up. Place, seam side down, in large baking pan.
Enchilada sauce, mild or hot	10 oz	Combine; pour over tortillas.
Tomato sauce	1 cup	
Cheddar cheese substitute	½ cup	Top with. Bake 25–30 minutes in 350F oven.
Nonfat yogurt	½ cup	Serve with.
Chopped cilantro	To taste	Serving size: 2 tortillas.

Nutrient Analysis

Calories	293
Total Fat	4.7 gr
Fiber	N/A
Cholesterol	36 mg

SOURCE: Robert Kowalski, *The 8-Week Cholesterol Cure Cookbook* (New York: Harper & Row, 1987).

Chicken and Rice

Ingredients	6 Portions	Method
Broiler-fryer chicken, 2½ lbs, cut up, skinned	1	Arrange chicken in roasting pan. Sauté onion in oil until transparent.
Green onions, sliced	½ cup	
Oil	½ tsp	
Chicken stock	2 cups	Add. Bake at 375F until mixture simmers; reduce heat to 250F. Bake for 1 hour or until chicken is tender.
Mushrooms, chopped	¾ cup	
Pimento, chopped	1 Tbsp	
Salt	To taste	
Pepper	To taste	
Rice, uncooked	1 cup	Steam until tender. Serve with chicken.
Plain, low-fat yogurt	½ cup	Use as garnish. Serving size: ⅙ chicken.

Nutrient Analysis

Calories	478
Total Fat	10.3 gr
Fiber	2 gr
Cholesterol	110 mg

SOURCE: Members of the American Dietetic Association. *Dietitians' Food Favorites.*

Refried Beans

Ingredients	6 Portions	Method
Olive oil	1 Tbsp	In large skillet, heat
Onion, chopped fine	¼ cup	oil. Add onion, garlic,
Garlic cloves, minced fine	2 large	and jalapeño pepper, and sauté for 2–3
Jalapeño pepper, minced fine	1	minutes.
Beans, red or pink	2 1-lb cans	Drain 1 can. Add contents of both cans to skillet (drained and undrained beans). Turn heat fairly high and mash beans with edge of wooden spoon until coarsely broken down. Reduce heat and simmer gently, stirring continuously with wooden spoon, 5–10 minutes, or until beans form coarse purée which begins to stick to bottom of skillet.
Lime juice	To taste	Season lightly with.
Cilantro, freshly chopped	To taste	Serving size: ⅙ recipe

Refried Beans   (Continued)

Nutrient Analysis

Calories	160
Total Fat	2.9 gr
Fiber	N/A
Cholesterol	0 mg

SOURCE: Kowalski, *The 8-Week Cholesterol Cure Cookbook.*

Now, see the differences on the following sample Advanced Heart Repair diet menus. The sample recipes allowed on the Advanced Heart Repair diet are so delicious that you may want to try them even if you are on the Basic Heart Maintenance diet.

ADVANCED HEART REPAIR DIET

Sample 1

BREAKFAST ⅓ cup **Prune Juice**
½ **Banana**
1 cup **Cream of Wheat**
1 teaspoon soft-tub **Margarine**
½ cup **Skim Milk**
Decaffeinated **Coffee** or **Tea**

LUNCH **Tossed Salad** (1 cup raw vegetables)
1 tablespoon **Fat-Free Dressing**
*½ cup **Broccoli-Noodle Bake**
1 slice **Whole Grain Bread**
*½ cup **Ambrosia Deluxe**
4 **Vanilla Wafers**
Decaffeinated **Coffee** or **Tea**

DINNER **Clams with Spaghetti** (3 oz clams, ⅔ cup
tomato sauce, 1 cup spaghetti)
1 **Dinner Roll**
½ cup **Skim Milk**
1 **Peach**
Decaffeinated **Coffee** or **Tea**

Broccoli-Noodle Bake

Ingredients	4 Portions	Method
Egg noodles, dry	4 oz	Cook noodles according to package directions.
Broccoli, chopped	¾ lb	Combine cooked noodles and broccoli.
Cottage cheese, low-fat (2% fat)	½ cup	Combine.
Egg substitute	¼ cup	
Oregano, ground	¼ tsp	
Garlic powder	⅛ tsp	
Pepper, black	Dash	
Cheddar cheese, grated	¼ cup	Combine half of the grated cheese with egg substitute mixture. Add broccoli/noodle mixture. Toss lightly. Pour into greased casserole. Top with remaining cheese. Bake at 350F for 30 minutes. Can substitute cauliflower for broccoli. Serving size: ½ cup.

Broccoli-Noodle Bake   (Continued)

Nutrient Analysis	
Calories	197
Total Fat	5.1 gr
Fiber	1.3 gr
Cholesterol	67 mg

SOURCE: Members of the American Dietetic Association. *Dietitians' Food Favorites.*

Ambrosia Deluxe

Ingredients	3 Portions	Method
Canned mandarin oranges, drained	5½ oz	Mix ingredients well. Refrigerate several hours
Canned pineapple chunks, drained	10 oz	before serving. Garnish with mint leaves or
Shredded coconut	2½ Tbsp	maraschino cherries.
Miniature marshmallows	¼ cup	Serving size: ½ cup.
Plain yogurt	¼ cup	

Nutrient Analysis

Calories	105
Total Fat	2.3 gr
Fiber	0.4 gr
Cholesterol	1 mg

SOURCE: Members of the American Dietetic Association. *Dietitians' Food Favorites.*

ADVANCED HEART REPAIR DIET

Sample 2

BREAKFAST   1 cup **Apple Juice**
1 cup **Oatmeal**
½ cup **Skim Milk**
1 teaspoon soft-tub **Margarine**
Decaffeinated **Coffee** or **Tea**

LUNCH   *1 cup **Pasta E Fagioli Soup**
6 unsalted **Crackers**
Vegetable Egg Substitute Omelette (½ cup
egg substitute, onions, mushrooms,
tomato—nonstick spray)
1 slice **Whole Wheat Bread**
1 **Peach**
Decaffeinated **Coffee** or **Tea**

DINNER   **Hearts of Lettuce Salad**
2 tablespoons fat-free **Dressing**
*4 ounces **Flounder Florentine**
1 **Sweet Potato**
½ cup **Stewed Tomatoes**
1 teaspoon soft-tub **Margarine**
½ cup **Skim Milk**
12 **Cherries**
Decaffeinated **Coffee** or **Tea**

Pasta E Fagioli (Pasta & Bean) Soup

Ingredients	4 Portions	Method
Olive oil	⅛ cup	Heat in large soup pot.
Large onion, pared, chopped	½	Add; cook over medium heat for 10 minutes.
Small green pepper, chopped	½	
Garlic clove, pared, minced	1	
Celery, chopped	¼ cup	
Carrot, pared, thinly sliced	½	
Italian-style tomatoes	7½ oz	Add; simmer for 15 minutes.
Parsley, chopped	⅛ cup	
Basil	½ tsp	
Condensed beef broth	1 10½ oz can	
Water	1 soup can	
Elbow or shell macaroni, uncooked	½ cup	Add; heat to boiling. Reduce heat; cook until tender.
Kidney beans	7½ oz	Add; heat for 10 minutes.
Parmesan cheese, grated	1 Tbsp	Sprinkle on before serving. Serving size: 1 cup.

Pasta E Fagioli (Pasta & Bean) Soup   (Continued)

Nutrient Analysis

Calories	155
Total Fat	4.4 gr
Fiber	6.7 gr
Cholesterol	9 mg

SOURCE: Members of the American Dietetic Association. *Dietitians' Food Favorites.*

Flounder Florentine

Ingredients	4 Portions	Method
Water	½ cup	Heat to boiling.
Frozen chopped spinach	1 10-oz pkg	Add; return water to boil, separating spinach with fork. Cover; cook for 2 minutes. Drain well.
Onion, pared, finely chopped	1 Tbsp	

Flounder Florentine (Continued)

Ingredients	4 Portions	Method
Marjoram	½ tsp	Add; combine. Place in glass baking dish.
Flounder fillets	1 lb	Arrange on spinach.
Skim milk Flour	1 cup 1 Tbsp	Combine flour with one quarter of milk. Heat remaining milk in saucepan. Add flour mixture; stir until thickened.
Pepper Nutmeg	Dash Dash	Stir into sauce; pour over fish.
Parmesan cheese, grated	2 Tbsp	Sprinkle over top. Bake at 400F for 25 minutes or until light brown and bubbly. Serving size: 4 oz.

Nutrient Analysis

Calories	147
Total Fat	2 gr
Fiber	1.4 gr
Cholesterol	60 mg

SOURCE: Members of the American Dietetic Association. *Dietitians' Food Favorites.*

A *Nutritional Survival Guide* 109

ADVANCED HEART REPAIR DIET

Sample 3

BREAKFAST 1 whole **Grapefruit**
1½ cups **Puffed Wheat Cereal**
½ cup **Skim Milk**
1 slice **Oatmeal Bread**
1 teaspoon soft-tub **Margarine**
Decaffeinated **Coffee** or **Tea**

LUNCH *¾ cup **Egg Drop Soup**
6 unsalted **Crackers**
Grilled Cheese on Rye with Tomato (2 oz
Alpine cheese, nonstick spray)
½ cup **Carrot Sticks**
1 cup **Applesauce**
1 slice **Angel Food Cake**
Decaffeinated **Coffee** or **Tea**

DINNER *3-inch by 3-inch **Vegetable Lasagna**
*½ cup **Marinated Coleslaw**
½ cup **Green Beans**
1 teaspoon soft-tub **Margarine**
1¼ cup **Strawberries** with ½ cup
Nonfat Vanilla Yogurt
Decaffeinated **Coffee** or **Tea**

Egg Drop Soup

Ingredients	4 Portions	Method
Condensed chicken broth	1 10½-oz can	Combine in saucepan; heat to
Water	1 soup can	boiling.
Cornstarch	1 Tbsp	Combine; stir into
Cold water	2 Tbsp	broth. Cook until slightly thickened.
Soy sauce	1 Tbsp	Stir in.
Green onions, sliced	2	
Egg, beaten	1	Stir in gently; remove from heat. Let stand for 1 minute before serving. Serving size: ¾ cup.

Nutrient Analysis

Calories	47
Total Fat	1.3 gr
Fiber	0.2 gr
Cholesterol	60 mg

SOURCE: Members of the American Dietetic Association. *Dietitians' Food Favorites.*

Vegetable Lasagna

Ingredients	4 Portions	Method
Tomato sauce	1½ cups	Combine.
Italian seasoning	⅛ tsp	
Garlic salt	¼ tsp	
Onion powder	¼ tsp	
Part-skim ricotta cheese	4 oz	Combine.
Low-fat cottage cheese	¼ cup	
Lasagna noodles, cooked	2 oz	Layer ½ in greased baking dish; layer ½ of cheese mixture.
Zucchini, unpared, uncooked, sliced	½	Layer ½ of each.
Fresh chopped spinach, thawed, drained	5 oz	
Part-skim mozzarella cheese, shredded	4 oz	Layer ½; layer ½ of tomato sauce. Repeat layers, topping with sauce and mozzarella. Bake at 325F for 30 minutes. Let cool for 10 minutes; serve. Serving size: 3″ by 3″ square.

Vegetable Lasagna   (Continued)

Nutrient Analysis

Calories	223
Total Fat	7.3 gr
Fiber	0.9 gr
Cholesterol	26 mg

SOURCE: Members of the American Dietetic Association. *Dietitians' Food Favorites.*

Marinated Coleslaw

Ingredients	3 Portions	Method
Cabbage, thinly sliced	½ lb	Mix together; let sit for 2 hours.
Salt	1 Tbsp	Drain; rinse thoroughly; drain.

Marinated Coleslaw (Continued)

Ingredients	3 Portions	Method
Carrot, pared, shredded	½	Add; reserve.
Green pepper, thinly sliced	¼	
Vinegar	¼ cup plus 2 tsp	Combine in
Sugar	¼ cup plus 2 Tbsp	saucepan; heat to
Dry mustard	½ tsp	boiling. Pour over
Hot pepper sauce	To taste	reserved cabbage
Water	¼ cup	mixture.
Mustard seed	⅛ tsp	Refrigerate
Celery seed	⅛ tsp	overnight; pour off liquid. Garnish with fresh parsley, dill, chervil, or coriander. Serving size: ½ cup.

Nutrient Analysis

Calories	77
Total Fat	0.3 gr
Fiber	1.2 gr
Cholesterol	0 mg

SOURCE: Members of the American Dietetic Association. *Dietitians' Food Favorites.*

ADVANCED HEART REPAIR DIET

Sample 4

BREAKFAST   1 cup **Orange Juice**
1 **English Muffin**
1 teaspoon soft-tub **Margarine**
½ cup **Skim Milk**
Decaffeinated **Coffee** or **Tea**

LUNCH   *1 cup **Marinated Vegetable Salad** mixed
with 1 cup **Kidney Beans**
1 slice **Whole Wheat Bread**
2 ounces unsalted **Pretzels**
2 **Tangerines**
Decaffeinated **Coffee** or **Tea**

DINNER   *¾ cup **Split Pea Soup**
*3 ounces **Sunshine Chicken Sesame**
*½ cup **Carrots à l'Orange**
*¾ cup **Ratatouille**
½ cup **Brown Rice**
1 cup canned **Peaches and Pears**
½ cup **Nonfat Frozen Yogurt**
Decaffeinated **Coffee** or **Tea**

Marinated Vegetable Salad

Ingredients	3 Portions	Method
Medium broccoli stalk, broken into florets	½	Combine all vegetables.
Small cauliflower head, broken into florets	½	
Large green pepper, cut into 1″ pieces	½	
Medium cucumber, sliced	½	
Medium carrots, pared, sliced	2	
Cherry tomatoes, stems removed	5	
Reduced-calorie Italian dressing	½ cup	Toss to coat. Cover; refrigerate overnight. Amounts and types of vegetables can be varied. Serving size: 1 cup.

Nutrient Analysis

Calories	80
Total Fat	0.6 gr
Fiber	2.8 gr
Cholesterol	0 mg

SOURCE: Members of the American Dietetic Association. *Dietitians' Food Favorites.*

Split Pea Soup

Ingredients	5 Portions	Method
Green split peas, dried, rinsed	½ lb	Cover peas with water and bring to boil.
Water	1¼ qt	Remove from heat; let stand for one hour.
Ham bone, meaty	1	Add; bring to boil.
Onion, pared, chopped	¾ cup	Cover, simmer at least 2 hours.
Black pepper	½ tsp	
Garlic salt	⅛ tsp	
Marjoram, dried	⅛ tsp	
Celery, diced	½ cup	Remove ham bone,
Carrots, pared, diced	½ cup	trim off and dice meat.
Parsley, fresh, minced	1 tsp	Discard bone. Add
Salt	To taste	ham and remaining ingredients. Cook slowly for about 45 minutes. Serve with minced parsley garnish, oyster crackers, or grated cheese.
		Serving size: ¾ cup.

Split Pea Soup   (Continued)

Nutrient Analysis

Calories	172
Total Fat	0.6 gr
Fiber	5.9 gr
Cholesterol	0 mg

SOURCE: Members of the American Dietetic Association. *Dietitians' Food Favorites.*

Sunshine Chicken Sesame

Ingredients	4 Portions	Method
Chicken breast halves, skinned	4	Season chicken; place on rack in roasting
Lemon pepper	To taste	pan.
Water	½ cup	Add. Cover; bake at 300F for 1 hour or until tender. Remove chicken; place on broiler pan.
Honey	¼ cup	Combine; brush on chicken. Broil 6 inches from heat until golden.
Frozen grapefruit concentrate, undiluted	2 Tbsp	
Sesame seeds	3 Tbsp	Top with. Serve with rice. Orange or lemon concentrate can be substituted for grapefruit. Serving size: 1 breast half.

Nutrient Analysis

Calories	259
Total Fat	6.6 gr
Fiber	0.3 gr
Cholesterol	73 mg

SOURCE: Members of the American Dietetic Association. *Dietitians' Food Favorites.*

Carrots à l'Orange

Ingredients	4 Portions	Method
Orange juice	½ cup	Heat to boiling.
Orange rind, grated	1 tsp	Add.
Lemon juice	1 tsp	
Cornstarch	1 tsp	Dissolve cornstarch in
Water	1 Tbsp	water. Add to orange mixture; heat, stirring, until thickened.
Medium-size carrots, pared, sliced	2	Steam until tender. Combine with thickened sauce; serve hot. Serving size: ½ carrot.

Nutrient Analysis

Calories	32
Total Fat	0.1 gr
Fiber	0.6 gr
Cholesterol	0 mg

SOURCE: Members of the American Dietetic Association. *Dietitians' Food Favorites.*

Ratatouille

Ingredients	5 Portions	Method
Whole tomatoes, cut into bite-size pieces	1 16-oz can	Combine in heavy saucepan; toss. Heat to boiling; reduce heat; simmer until fork-tender.
Zucchini, cut lengthwise in quarters, seeded, core removed; cut into bit-size pieces	1 cup	
Eggplant, pared, cut into 1″ cubes	1 cup	
Small bell pepper, sliced	½	
Small red onion, pared, thinly sliced	½	
Oregano	1½ tsp	
Parsley, chopped	1½ tsp	
Garlic clove, pared, crushed	1	
Black pepper	Pinch	
Salt substitute	As desired	Taste and adjust seasonings; better when held and reheated.
Artificial sweetener	As desired	Serving size: ⅔ cup.

Ratatouille　(Continued)

Nutrient Analysis	
Calories	41
Total Fat	0.4 gr
Fiber	1.3 gr
Cholesterol	0 mg

SOURCE: Members of the American Dietetic Association. *Dietitians' Food Favorites.*

ADVANCED HEART REPAIR DIET

Sample 5

BREAKFAST 1 cup **Orange Juice**
2 slices **Wheat Toast**
1 teaspoon soft-tub **Margarine**
½ cup **Skim Milk**
Decaffeinated **Coffee** or **Tea**

LUNCH *1 cup (⅙ recipe) **Black Bean Chili Soup**
*1 slice **Yogurt Cornbread**
1 **Whole Wheat Pita**
1 cup **Fresh Fruit Cup**
Decaffeinated **Coffee** or **Tea**

DINNER *¾ cup **Enchilada Bake**
½ cup **Steamed Rice**
Tossed Salad with 1 tablespoon **Fat-Free Dressing**
1 teaspoon soft-tub **Margarine**
½ cup **Nonfat Plain Yogurt** topped with **Banana**
Decaffeinated **Coffee** or **Tea**

Black Bean Chili Soup
Susan E. Slesinger, Lakewood, CA

Ingredients	8 Portions	Method
Black turtle beans (*frijoles negros*), uncooked, rinsed Water	12 oz	Combine beans with enough water to cover by 2 inches.
Olive oil	2 Tbsp plus 2 tsp	In 4-qt saucepan
Onions, chopped	2 cups	heat oil over
Green chili pepper, seeded, chopped	2 Tbsp	medium heat; add onions, chili
Garlic cloves, minced	6	pepper, garlic, and sauté, stirring
Water	1 qt. plus 3 cups	occasionally, until
Italian tomatoes, canned (with liquid), drained, seeded, and diced, reserving liquid	2 cups	onions are softened. Drain beans; add to saucepan along with water and remaining
Cumin, ground	2 tsp	ingredients except
Chili powder	1 tsp	yogurt; mix well;
Coriander, ground	1 tsp	bring to boil.
Red pepper, crushed	½ tsp	Reduce heat to low, cover pan, and let simmer, stirring occasionally, until beans are tender, about 2 hours.

Black Bean Chili Soup (Continued)

Ingredients	8 Portions	Method
		Remove from heat; let cool. Pour 1–2 cups at a time into blender and process until smooth, until half the soup is processed. Pour soup back into saucepan with unprocessed soup and cook over medium heat until heated through, 5–10 minutes.
Yogurt, plain, low-fat	2 cups	Top with, ¼ cup per serving. Serving size: ⅛ finished recipe.

Nutrient Analysis

Calories	253
Total Fat	6 gr
Fiber	N/A
Cholesterol	3 mg

SOURCE: *Weight Watchers Favorite Recipes: Over 280 Winning Dishes from Weight Watchers Members and Staff* (New York: NAL-Dutton, 1986).

Yogurt Cornbread

Ingredients	4 Portions	Method
Vegetable oil	1 Tbsp plus 1 tsp	In baking pan, heat oil at 400F for about 2 minutes.
White cornmeal mix, uncooked, self-rising	3 oz	Combine all but 1 tsp cornmeal, flour, sugar, baking soda and, if desired, salt; stir in yogurt. Remove pan from oven. Pour hot oil into cornmeal mixture; stir to combine. Sprinkle remaining tsp cornmeal over bottom of pan; spoon in cornmeal mixture. Bake at 400F until golden brown, 25–30 minutes. Serve hot. Serving size: ¼ of cornbread.
Flour, self-rising	1 Tbsp plus 1 tsp	
Sugar, granulated	1½ tsp	
Baking soda	1 tsp	
Salt (optional)	Dash	
Yogurt, plain, low-fat	1 cup	

Yogurt Cornbread   (Continued)

Nutrient Analysis

Calories	165
Total Fat	6 gr
Fiber	N/A
Cholesterol	3 mg

SOURCE: *Weight Watchers Favorite Recipes: Over 280 Winning Dishes from Weight Watchers Members and Staff.*

Enchilada Bake

Ingredients	6 Portions	Method
Medium onion, pared, chopped	1	Sauté until onion is translucent.
Green pepper, chopped	1	
Sliced mushrooms, drained	1 4-oz can	
Garlic clove, pared, minced	1	
Dry pinto beans	½ cup	Cook according to package directions. Drain; add.

Enchilada Bake (Continued)

Ingredients	6 Portions	Method
Stewed tomatoes	1½ cups	Add; combine.
Chili powder	1 Tbsp	Simmer over low heat
Ground cumin	1 tsp	for 30 minutes.
Salt	½ tsp	
Corn tortillas	6	Arrange half in oiled casserole. Cover with half of bean mixture.
Monterey Jack cheese, shredded	½ cup	Sprinkle half over bean mixture.
Ricotta cheese, part-skim	¼ cup	Combine; spoon half over Jack cheese.
Yogurt, plain, low-fat	¼ cup	Repeat layers, reserving enough bean sauce to top off casserole. Bake at 350F for 15–20 minutes. Garnish with ripe olives. Serving size: ¾ cup.

Nutrient Analysis

Calories	252
Total Fat	5.4 gr
Fiber	1.3 gr
Cholesterol	11 mg

SOURCE: Members of the American Dietetic Association. *Dietitians' Food Favorites.*

Checkpoint 1 — *Six-Week Evaluation*

When the first CVI orientation group reached the six-week evaluation point, we asked all the members how they felt they were doing, and whether or not they were comfortable with the program. Let's take a look to see how the five group members we're following were doing in their countdowns toward zero.

MARIE CORELLI, on the Basic Heart Maintenance diet with fiber supplement (psyllium), managed after six weeks to bring her LDL down only to 190. Her HDL had stayed the same, too low at 40. Steve put her on the Advanced Heart Repair diet and continued the supplemental fiber. She had not been able to stop smoking, or even to cut down, which was not helping her raise her HDL, and although she'd chosen swimming as her form of exercise, she was still not swimming long enough or hard enough to be of benefit in reversing her atherosclerosis (or raising her HDL either). However, she felt there was enough improvement there to rate herself a 2. Because she still worried about finances and her health, and was experiencing emotional problems, her stress score of 2⅔ remained the same, despite relaxation exercises. Her score was still high risk at six weeks.

She told Steve she was pinning all her hopes on the program.

Marie's Score:

$$\left[\frac{LDL}{10} - \frac{HDL}{5}\right] + 2\left[\begin{array}{c}\text{\# OF PACKS}\\\text{PER DAY}\end{array}\right] + \begin{array}{c}\text{EXERCISE}\\\text{SCORE}\end{array} + \begin{array}{c}\text{STRESS}\\\text{SCORE}\end{array} + \frac{SBP - 130}{20} = \underline{\quad}$$

$$[\ 19\ -\ 8\ ] +\quad 4\quad +\quad 2\quad +\ 2\frac{2}{3}\ +\quad 0\quad = 19\frac{2}{3}$$

CARLA PETERS was ecstatic. Her LDL had dropped from 196 to 150, and her HDL had risen from 40 to our basic target of at least 50. Her exercise score dropped to 2, and in redoing her stress test she realized she was sleeping better, felt less hostile toward the people around her, and less like she had insurmountable health problems, cutting her score in half from its original 2, down to 1. She'd already dropped from high risk to medium risk in only six weeks, and she said, rather tentatively, that she was starting to feel more comfortable around some of her classmates.

I had her continue on the Basic Heart Maintenance diet.

Carla's Score:

$$\left[\frac{LDL}{10} - \frac{HDL}{5}\right] + 2\left[\begin{array}{c}\text{\# OF PACKS}\\\text{PER DAY}\end{array}\right] + \begin{array}{c}\text{EXERCISE}\\\text{SCORE}\end{array} + \begin{array}{c}\text{STRESS}\\\text{SCORE}\end{array} + \frac{SBP - 130}{20} = \underline{\quad}$$

$$[\ 15\ -\ 10\ ] +\quad 0\quad +\quad 2\quad +\ 1\ +\quad 1\quad = 9$$

ED DONALDSON had a heart attack and died. I don't mean to state it that baldly, but there's really no easy way to say it. It happened about a month into the program. He would have had little change in his numbers since he was doing nothing about them. Up until the day of his death, it must be assumed that his scores were the same, including his blood pressure, for he refused to take any medication, despite the fact that we repeatedly stressed the importance of his full cooperation if the program was to have any effect.

FRANK KELSEY was overjoyed with his early progress. His LDL had fallen from 170 to 135, and his HDL, already at an acceptable level, was up slightly, from 50 to 52. He was exercising faithfully and his score had dropped to 2. His stress score, which was originally 1, was now counted down to 0. Best of all, his blood pressure was normal for the first time in years on his new regimen of diet—now including lots of fish—and exercise. His score had dropped from moderately high risk to medium risk in only six weeks, and he was becoming something of a group cheerleader.

I had him continue on the Basic Heart Maintenance diet.

Frank's Score:

$$\left[\frac{LDL}{10} - \frac{HDL}{5} \right] + 2\left[\begin{array}{c} \# \text{ OF PACKS} \\ \text{PER DAY} \end{array} \right] + \begin{array}{c} \text{EXERCISE} \\ \text{SCORE} \end{array} + \begin{array}{c} \text{STRESS} \\ \text{SCORE} \end{array} + \frac{SBP - 130}{20} = \underline{\quad}$$

$$[\ 14\ -\ 10\ ] + \qquad 0 \quad + \quad 2 \quad + \quad 0 \quad + \quad 0 \quad = 6$$

TONY SPAGNOLA had a slight drop in his LDL, from 111 to 107—very good. But his HDL remained very low at 25. He had cut his 1 pack of cigarettes a day down to half a pack, and said he'd done so without much trouble, so it was hopeful his HDL would start rising if he quit smoking entirely. His exercise score began at and remained at 1. Stress was still 1⅓.

Tony's classmates all seemed to feel relaxed around him; he apparently liked everyone equally, and wanted badly to succeed.

Steve added psyllium to Tony's diet to push his LDL to 100,

and again told him that he must stop smoking completely for the exercise to have any effect on his HDL. His score had dropped from barely above medium risk to the definite medium range.

Tony's Score:

$$\left[\frac{LDL}{10} - \frac{HDL}{5}\right] + 2\left[\begin{array}{c}\text{\# OF PACKS} \\ \text{PER DAY}\end{array}\right] + \begin{array}{c}\text{EXERCISE} \\ \text{SCORE}\end{array} + \begin{array}{c}\text{STRESS} \\ \text{SCORE}\end{array} + \frac{SBP - 130}{20} = \underline{\quad}$$

$$[\ 11\ -\ 5\ ] +\quad 1\quad +\quad 1\quad +\quad 1\frac{1}{3}\ +\quad 0\quad = 9\frac{1}{3}$$

How are *you* doing, six weeks into the program? Did you enter your new numbers on the six-week sheets at the back of the book? Are you getting a little closer to zero?

4 *The Exercise High*

South Philadelphia has spawned great sports stars. Two of my friends and patients—Joey Giardello and Joe Frazier—are prime examples. Unfortunately, love of sport, as translated into love of exercise, doesn't seem to be the norm for the majority of people.

At the session on exercise, a couple of our class members told me that they'd visited the gym to use the equipment. But most admitted they hadn't been to our gym or done anything else in the way of starting an exercise program to bring their exercise scores toward zero. I wish I could say I was surprised, but I wasn't. It's nothing new—this aversion so many people show to sweating.

Do you feel the same way? Why? Do you have any idea how much better you feel when you exercise? I exercise. Steve exercises. It's not always the same exercise and not every day. We don't have time. But I know for myself that if I didn't exercise at least three times a week, this is what I'd feel like. I'd be lethargic. I wouldn't have enough energy to do all the things my job and life require. I'd always be telling myself I'd get started tomorrow, or next week, or right after New Year's—one excuse after another. I'd find myself gaining weight over the years, and I'd excuse myself on the grounds that everyone gains weight as they get older. (By the way, that doesn't have to be true.) And all the while, the lethargy would continue to envelop every thought, every desire and attitude.

I'd no longer sleep as well as I did when I was younger. My sex life would be less satisfying. I wouldn't enjoy eating as much, because my digestion would be poorer. My skin would start to look sort of grayish, but I'd say that was age, too. The healthy flush of youth was lost to me, but what could I do?

Well, that's all garbage. I'll tell you what I could do in those circumstances. It's what I expect you to do to improve your entire outlook, your way of life, your tolerance, your zest.

Exercise! The only thing difficult about exercising is the enormous effort many people put into finding reasons why they don't want to start.

Think about when you were a child. You ran around and played games. You didn't stop and think about the fact that you were exercising, you just did it. You took part in activities that got your heart pumping and your blood surging through your body. That got your appetite up, you enjoyed eating, and yet didn't ever gain an ounce of weight.

Well, your body still needs activity like that, no matter what age you've attained. We're animals. We have muscles that need flexing and strengthening. When things go unused, they deteriorate. We get flabby, we get cranky. We want to do less and less. Slow down enough and we even lose our natural desire to see what the next day has in store for us.

All this happens because our brains need the sense of our bodies working. When we exercise, we feel sharper, problem solving is easier. Nothing seems beyond our capacity.

Our patients who finally make a commitment to regular exercise tell us with surprise that nothing feels better than working up a sweat. Nothing makes them feel younger than getting their muscles toned up. Skin tightening. Breathing deep breaths of life. They are obviously astonished to admit that all sorts of physical activity, from jogging, bicycling, and swimming to rope jumping, push-ups, sit-ups, create the greatest high in the world.

And it's true. I know it for a fact. It's what keeps Steve and me going under impossibly heavy workloads. It's what makes us keep setting new goals and looking for new worlds to conquer.

There are two basic types of exercise, and both will improve your life. One is *static* (such as moving heavy objects and formal weightlifting). The other is *dynamic* (aerobic), which describes all those in this chapter, because it's the aerobic type of exercise, done regularly, that protects against coronary heart disease. Many exercises are a combination of both types. Tennis is a good example. But most exercises are predominantly one or the other.

If you recall, I explained to you back in the Introduction why aerobic exercise is good for your heart. To summarize:

Aerobic exercise increases the size of your coronary arteries, creating larger openings through which the blood can flow; promotes the development of collaterals—natural bypasses that form gradually, in response to blocked arteries, to deliver blood to undernourished areas of the heart muscle (and good collaterals can prevent a heart attack or limit its consequences); reduces the tendency of your blood platelets to clump, decreasing the risk of clot formation. Even if a clot should form, such exercise enhances your body's own clot-dissolving mechanisms.

Furthermore, when you and I exercise regularly, we benefit in these additional ways:

- Lower blood pressure—expect a 10-point drop in systolic and diastolic pressure even with moderate levels of regular exercise;
- Higher HDL—with a moderate aerobic exercise program,

we can anticipate, over a six- to twelve-month period, a 10 percent increase, which seems to occur even without weight loss or a change in diet;

* Less body fat, leading to lower LDL and triglycerides;
* Are you a diabetic? Physical activity enhances the body's ability to extract glucose from the blood, thereby reducing blood sugar levels;
* Are you a smoker? Exercise makes quitting easier;
* Stress reduction—we have a natural fight-or-flight response to stress, which I'll discuss in Chapter 5. For now, let me just say that fight-or-flight is accommodated safely by exercise, which really puts our bodies in gear;
* Are you overweight? You'll have an easier time losing those pounds. This is a proven fact. Aerobic exercise speeds up the metabolism for continued burning of calories hours after the activity ends. More than 34 million Americans are obese, like Carla—20 percent or more above their ideal range of body weight. It appears that obesity is more closely tied to low energy output than to caloric intake. It's characterized by a sedentary lifestyle, an increase in LDL, a decrease in HDL, and elevated fasting triglycerides (your blood test number for triglycerides on an empty stomach). If you feel you're overweight, even by just a few pounds, you'll be amazed at what exercise can do not only for your waistline but for your entire body.

In all these ways, exercise can lengthen and enhance your life. The risk to your heart if you're too lazy to exercise is on the same order of magnitude as the risk of high blood pressure, high cholesterol, and smoking. When all the available studies of the link between exercise and heart disease are analyzed, it's estimated that inactive people are nearly twice as likely to die of a heart attack as active people, even after adjusting for other risk factors.

And yet, despite the supposed popularity of activities like jogging and bicycling, 60 percent of American adults don't get enough exercise. Instead, the tendency is toward slowing down and also toward obesity. This translates into millions of people at risk.

Which category are you in? Which do you *want* to be in: the category for those who enjoy life, or for those who avoid living life as much as possible? Well, it's time to do something about it.

The first thing I want you to do, if you've been putting it off, is to have that exercise stress test. This is very important, especially if you have already been diagnosed as having heart disease. The stress test will not only uncover any potential problems, but will also enable the physician monitoring you to tell you what your training zone is. The value of aerobic exercise is that it keeps your heart within this training zone, which allows the best results in reversing atherosclerosis.

Once you know your own training zone, you will know what your pulse rate should be, taken during and/or after exercise. Now you can decide what kind of exercise best suits you. Just give it some thought. Are you a swimmer? Do you like jogging? Bicycling? Or do you like walking, or a combination of walking and jogging: power walking?

What activity gets your blood surging and gives you an incredible high? And don't tell me, no activity. I expect you to do better than that, not only for the sake of your circulatory system but for the sake of your entire quality of life.

A minimum of 20 minutes (depending on the type of exercise you choose) will be necessary to keep your metabolic rate accelerated for up to six hours after the end of the exercise period. And that's good for your digestion and for continued burn-off of calories.

Okay. Let's assume you've had your stress test and been given the go-ahead to start your exercise program. You've been told what your pulse rate should be to keep your heart rate within the training zone.

Now for the part that's momentous, for this is another step you're taking to control your own destiny: Choosing your type of exercise.

The exercises described in the following pages are all aerobic. Remember, aerobic exercises promote regression of atherosclerosis, which is the ultimate goal of the Philadelphia Formula. But don't overlook other, gentler forms of exercise, from playing golf (without using a golf cart to take you from hole to hole) to the simple up and down, bending and stretching of gardening.

All of these activities will enhance your life

When doing the exercises that follow, be sure to spend at least five minutes before each exercise session warming up (calisthenics and stretching exercises are good), and another five minutes after you exercise cooling down, to prevent muscle tightness, which causes pain, stiffness, and soreness.

In general, unless I've otherwise indicated, plan on at least three sessions a week.

The Walk-Jog Options

These are great choices if you have low exercise tolerance, weakened heart muscle, anginal chest pain, or bad arthritis, because you're better off with lower-intensity exercise done over a longer period of time. Don't overdo it. Start slowly and build up.

Table 7 shows a nine-step walking program that eventually works up to a four-mile-per-hour brisk walk. Frank initially chose this activity, which was wise, for remember, he was experiencing chest pains with any type of activity. Later, as he got into better shape, he alternated between brisk walking and stationary cycling.

Table 8 shows a walk-jog program where you gauge your walking speed by covering a fixed distance within an allotted time span.

Table 7
Nine-Step Walk Program

During Week #	Activity	Distance (*miles*)	Time Goal (*minutes*)
1	Walk	2.00	60
2	Walk	2.25	60
3	Walk	2.50	60
4	Walk	2.75	60
5	Walk	3.00	60
6	Walk	3.25	60
7	Walk	3.50	60
8	Brisk walk	3.75	60
9	Brisk walk	4.00	60

Remember, when doing all of these exercises, *take the time to warm up and to cool down*. It can make the difference between success in your efforts and failure due to aching muscles, leading to a desire to simply quit. Don't do that to yourself. Give yourself every chance for a full and active life.

Bicycling

Stationary cycling can be done for 20-minute sessions once you've slowly worked up, conditioning your muscles and increasing your stamina (see Table 9).

Resistance should be adjusted so that your pulse rate, counted for 15 seconds immediately after completing the exercise, then multiplied by 4, is within your target heart rate zone, explained to you by your doctor. As I mentioned, Frank went on to enjoy this form of exercise.

One of our class members took me aside at our session on exercise. He said that he and Carla were using stationary bikes at the gym at CVI. I'm including the basics of that conversation here, because I want to make a point about obesity. He said:

Table 8

Walk-Jog Program

Week	Activity	Distance (*miles*)	Time Goal (*minutes*)	Speed (*miles per hour*)
1	Walk	2.00	45	2.67
2	Walk	2.00	40	3.00
3	Walk	2.00	35	3.45
4	Walk	2.50	42	3.57
5	Walk	3.00	50	3.61
6	Brisk walk	3.00	45	4.00
7	Walk/Jog	2.00	28	4.26
8	Jog	2.00	26	4.65
9	Jog	2.00	23	5.26
10	Jog	2.50	27	5.56

"I was stunned to see Carla come into the gym this afternoon. So you're thinking, what's the big deal? It's just that I usually come much later myself, so I never saw Carla here before.

"Anyway, I was surprised. I was into my own exercising so I was breathing kind of hard, and to sort of distract myself from my own huffing and puffing, which irritates me, I started asking myself why I was so surprised to see her in a gym

"I figured, face it, she isn't the type. And thinking that, I got real angry at myself. Because I don't even know what type she is. I've never talked to her to get to know her better. She's real shy.

"I think maybe I was judging her on just the fact she's overweight. That must be it, since that's all I know about her. But I'm in a gym and I'm overweight, so why am I surprised and who am I to talk? I always figured I'd never laugh at anybody because of how they look or what they are.

"I'm disgusted with myself."

The point I want to make is this. Many people find them-

Table 9

Stationary Bicycle: Exercise Program

Step	Speed (*miles per hour*)	Time Goal (*minutes*)	Pulse Rate (*after exercise*)
1	15	4	Target Heart Rate
2	15	7	Target Heart Rate
3	15	10	Target Heart Rate
4	15	13	Target Heart Rate
5	17.5/65	16	Target Heart Rate
6	17.5/65	19	Target Heart Rate
7	17.5/65	22	Target Heart Rate
8	20/25	23	Target Heart Rate
9	20/75	24	Target Heart Rate
10	25/90	25	Target Heart Rate

selves thinking that way about someone obese. That's all they see. Often, they laugh about it to themselves or comment on it to friends.

But obesity is no laughing matter. It's associated with an increased risk of high blood pressure, abnormal lipid profile, heart failure, diabetes, and sudden death. Mild to moderate obesity doubles the risk of coronary disease. Severe obesity triples it. Obesity is also associated with an overall higher death rate for both men and women and is a powerful risk factor in younger patients.

For example, a twenty-five to thirty-four-year-old who is obese has a 50 percent higher risk of death from all causes than someone of normal weight of the same age and sex. Preventing obesity in childhood may be the most important factor in preventing abnormalities of blood lipids later in life.

Losing weight is a slow and tedious business, but combining exercise with diet strengthens your muscles while you burn off fat and accelerates the entire process. Oh, and by the way, recent studies indicate that fat distribution plays a role in predicting coronary risk. Heart disease is more common in big-bellied men and women than in their counterparts whose excess weight is carried further below the waist (hips, thighs, buttocks, etc.).

Enough about losing weight. I've got four more aerobic exercises to recommend to you.

Outdoor Cycling

Outdoor cycling is very enjoyable. Just remember, you should normally wear a helmet. If you maintain an average speed of about 15 mph, you can achieve a good training effect. Higher speeds can be safely used with proper supervision and instruction.

Tony chose outdoor cycling.

Rope Jumping

This exercise rhythmically uses large muscle groups and keeps the heart rate raised over prolonged periods. It does take coordination so, as with any exercise, start slowly.

Aerobic Dancing

This is an excellent means of sustaining an accelerated heart rate. Three or four 30- to 40-minute sessions a week are necessary. The obvious drawback is the need for a qualified instructor.

Swimming

I really recommend swimming. It's outstanding for the cardiovascular and respiratory systems, because it keeps the heart rate elevated for sustained periods by the rhythmic use of upper and lower body muscles.

It is also very relaxing. This is obviously an enormously important point. And there are relatively fewer injuries than in other forms of exercise because of the cushioning effect of the water.

If you choose swimming, plan on two to three sessions a week, each lasting at least 30 minutes in water around 70 degrees. Very warm water should be avoided. The crawl and back strokes are the most beneficial.

Marie chose swimming.

What was your choice? Have you stuck to it? If you have, you're feeling remarkably livelier, aren't you? No shortness of breath climbing steps? Sleeping well? Generally happier all around, with the ups and downs of life assuming their proper proportions?

The exercise high should be helping you not only to bring your exercise risk factor score toward zero, but in your efforts at stress reduction as well.

5 The Relaxation Response— Easing Down

Carla Peters and two other members of the first orientation group were from South Philadelphia. One of them was the oldest member of the group, a seventy-nine-year-old woman. Steve and I have since met many members of their large families, which are typical of a majority of the families in South Philadelphia. These individuals are full of personality, laugh hard, and do everything to excess. Most important, they abound in those vital traits that make them strong: concern with religion, commitment to family, and throughout the family, intense loyalty.

I've often walked into a South Philadelphia hospital in the middle of the night to go to the aid of a heart attack victim, and found twenty to thirty highly emotional relatives crowded into the waiting room, keeping vigil. The men are never ashamed to hug and kiss each other for comfort, or to cry over the joys and sorrows of life.

At the session on stress, our seventy-nine-year-old's seat was empty. She'd suffered a heart attack the day before. She had some underlying heart disease but none of her arteries was completely blocked and her heart muscle was intact.

What happened was this: She'd had a shock crossing the street. Because she was partially deaf, she failed to hear an ambulance approaching. She was nearly hit, and in that moment of terror, of screeching brakes, her mind couldn't immediately grasp what was happening, and the areas of her heart muscle that were supplied by the partially blocked arteries became oxygen-starved. This made her heart electrically unstable.

An erratic rhythm began. Her heart's ability to function as a pump was disrupted. With the blood supply cut off to the brain and other vital organs, death would have been inevitable if the ambulance personnel had not been available and able to abort the lethal rhythm.

She was very lucky.

Steve and I both visited her in the hospital. All things considered, she was in far better spirits than many of her relatives.

This wasn't her first episode. She'd had a silent heart attack in the past (a heart attack that occurs without pain, and is revealed only on an electrocardiogram). This time she'd almost been a victim of one of the biggest potential killers of adults in the United States—sudden cardiac death syndrome. An electrical storm short-circuits the heart's normal pacemaker capability, resulting in an unstable rhythm called *ventricular fibrillation.*

As I say, she was very lucky. I've seen all too often how stress affects the heart. Over the long term, stress affects the development of coronary heart disease. That's why stress reduction is part of the Philadelphia Formula, and why bringing your stress risk factor score toward zero is so important.

Anger, fear, grief, or intense joy are all natural, daily reactions to stress, though I know it's difficult to conceive of joy or excitement as being stressful. All these emotions trigger our fight-or-flight response, a basic instinct inherited from our animal forebears and meant to prepare us to either fight or flee in dangerous situations.

Fight-or-flight can cause the brain to release hormones called *catecholamines,* one of which is adrenaline. Because this response is so rarely needed in today's world, it poses a potential danger. It makes the heart pound faster and harder, raising blood pressure. If constricted coronary arteries or scar tissue from a previous heart attack are present, some regions of the heart muscle may not be able to meet the higher oxygen demands of such stimulation.

Stress can be a deadly thing. Aside from its direct effect on the heart, stress also has significant effects on the blood. When we're anxious, fearful, angry, or hostile, clotting time is shortened. The blood becomes more viscous, more syrupy. Nature may have intended these adaptations to prevent major blood loss if fight-or-flight resulted in bleeding wounds, but without the actual fight-or-flight, such changes make undesirable clot formation more likely. When unwanted clots occur inside coronary arteries, the result can be an acute heart attack.

Chronic stress—for example, job-related stress—can be insidious and deadly. It causes levels of the anti-inflammatory hormone cortison (produced by the adrenal glands) to rise, and disproportionate levels of cortisone have been linked to diabetes and atherosclerosis. Stress-related surges in adrenaline can make the heartbeat electrically unstable and cause sudden cardiac death.

It's difficult these days not to lead a stressful life. But would you know if you were under an *abnormal* degree of stress, or would you simply regard the way you feel as normal? If you've done the simple stress evaluation at the end of the book (see Appendix C) to calculate your stress score, you've taken the first step toward dealing with this risk factor for coronary heart disease. The next step is working to bring that starting score toward zero. Had you made any progress in that direction when you redid your score at the six-week checkpoint?

Many coronary-prone patients are worriers or joyless strivers, and more significantly, they frequently suppress their anger. Some fit the Type A personality, which has become an icon of popular culture: the competitive, hard-driving man or woman on the fast track, under pressure to get things done yesterday, who eventually drops dead of a fatal heart attack.

Of the many factors known to cause heart-damaging stress, chronic occupational stress stands out most clearly (although in this area, as in others we've discussed, you can be sure there are dissenting studies). It not only contributes to heart attacks and sudden cardiac death but also fosters the progression of atherosclerosis. If you have little control over your work environment, you may experience significant mental stress, coupled with no corresponding outlet of physical energy. This brings on the fight-or-flight mechanism, with no counterbalance available. A situation is created whereby catecholamines are excreted unnecessarily and over a prolonged period into the bloodstream, elevating blood pressure and lipid levels. Fibrinogen levels may also rise, increasing the tendency of the blood to clot.

A job that includes time restraints and time pressure, boredom, lack of control, excessive noise, poor relations with management, and ambiguity will contribute to occupational stress. Does this sound like you, in your particular work environment?

Of all the members of the class, this was most clearly Tony's problem. At the time of the orientation, he'd been a construction worker for fourteen years, and a construction foreman for the last two. Then a new project came along, and he started coming home each night feeling tired and sick. It was a really big job in center city, and had to be finished in six months. As if that wasn't bad enough, Tony was given a skeleton crew of young, relatively inexperienced men to work with.

The real stress problem? The responsibility was all his, yet he had little control. He started to feel his heart pounding constantly and his face getting red. He was unable to get a good night's sleep. With the project only a month from its completion deadline, Tony had a heart attack.

Occupational stress—for many people just like Tony, you, and me—is so dire for the cardiovascular system because it occurs daily, repetitively, and chronically. Recognizing it and learning how to cope with it may add years to your life and save you from the ravages of atherosclerosis.

Here's what I do about it.

First of all, I try to pace myself. You must try to do this, too. Stop telling yourself what should have been done yesterday. Try to prepare well in advance for major life changes you know are coming. Planning for them will help keep them from becoming so stressful you can't confront them. Take as much time as possible in arriving at decisions, so you can think out different ways to adjust to actual events. And when reviewing your accomplishments, avoid viewing them as a time to screech to a dead halt. Life isn't like that. It's vital to continue striving, to find new goals.

Most important, I want to help you learn how to relax. The most obvious ways of doing this are by taking vacations or just occasional days off, little holidays on weekends when you do nothing but relax, a night out bowling . . . You'll be able to come up with a wealth of possibilities.

Of course, there are specific stress reduction techniques to help you achieve the often difficult goal of actually easing down. The need to ease down is vital, for relaxation is a natural enemy of the fight-or-flight mechanism.

Stress manifests itself in anger and inner hostility, backaches, fears and apprehensions, headaches, palpitations, hyperventilation, dizziness not brought on by organic problems, insomnia and sleeping abnormalities, chronic constipation and diarrhea, eating compulsion or anorexia, and obsessions. Take a few minutes now to evaluate how you feel, and if you're experiencing such feelings of stress, try the following easy relaxation technique:

Sit in a quiet room with as few distractions as possible. Shift your mind away from external worrying thoughts. To accomplish this, you'll find it helpful to silently repeat a sound, word, or phrase (called a *mantra*), or to gaze fixedly at an object you find pleasing.

Don't worry if distracting thoughts still occur. Try not to worry yourself over anything. Be sure you're comfortable. It's best not to actually lie down unless you're preparing for a nap or for bed at night, because as you really relax you may fall asleep.

Perform this relaxation exercise for five minutes every morning before you start your day. It's a very small commitment for something so good for you, physically and mentally. Done faithfully, you're sure to find your stress risk factor score moving closer to zero.

There are many formal techniques for evoking the same physiological outcome. A small sampling includes biofeedback (which uses electronic instruments to gauge the body's response to stress); meditation (which in effect winds down the sympathetic nervous system, resulting in lower heart and respiratory rates); hypnosis (which is essentially a state of enhanced suggestibility); massage (which has its roots in Chinese medicine, but which cannot, for the most part, be effectively practiced alone); and a method quite a few of my friends and patients seem to like—Progressive Relaxation, which uses the ability of voluntary skeletal muscles to relax. I've been told that this seems a more natural method of stress reduction than some of the more formalized types, such as yoga.

Let me briefly explain what is required in Progressive Relaxation. The idea behind this technique is that alternately contracting and releasing a muscle leads to progressively improved relaxation. Mentally focusing on the difference between the tensed and relaxed states promotes ever lower levels of tension. During this process, you can identify specific muscle groups suffering from chronic tension. The method requires a quiet room and lying prone—minimizing external factors that can lead to even the slightest measurable increases in muscle tension.

For an example of the Progressive Relaxation technique, assume a relaxed position. Make a fist with your right hand and tighten your grip as much as possible. Maintaining the clenched position, observe the sensation in the fist, hand, and forearm. When this can no longer be maintained, relax the closed fist quickly. Sense the limpness in your right hand and try to appreciate how it differs from the tension you previously felt. Repeat the exercise again and again, concentrating on the fact that relaxation is diametrically opposed to tension. Then go on to carry out the entire ritual with your left fist, and then with both fists simultaneously.

Other exercises involve other muscle groups. Similar results can be achieved with exercises concentrating on the head, chest, stomach, lower back, thighs, buttocks, calves, and feet. If you'd like to give it a try to see if it's right for you, the following series of exercises should last about 15 minutes:

1. Curl toes tightly. Hold. Relax. Rest.
2. Flex the feet. Hold. Relax. Rest.
3. Tighten the calves. Hold. Relax. Rest.
4. Tense the thighs. Hold. Relax. Rest.
5. Tighten the buttocks. Hold. Relax. Rest.
6. Tighten the lower back. Hold. Relax. Rest.
7. Tighten the abdomen. Hold. Relax. Rest.
8. Tighten the upper chest. Hold. Relax. Rest.
9. Tense the upper back muscles. Hold. Relax. Rest.
10. Clench the fists. Hold. Relax. Rest.
11. Extend the fingers and flex the wrists. Hold. Relax. Rest.
12. Tighten the forearms. Hold. Relax. Rest.
13. Tighten the upper arms. Hold. Relax. Rest.
14. Lift the shoulders gently toward the ears. Hold. Let them drop. Rest.
15. Wrinkle the forehead. Hold. Relax. Rest.
16. Squeeze your eyes shut. Hold. Relax. Rest.

17. Drop your chin, letting your mouth open widely. Hold. Relax. Rest.
18. Lift the shoulders gently and then pull them down as if you had weights in your hands. Rest.

Well—how do you feel? In the Suggested Readings and Selected References, Steve and I will direct you to several books detailing other relaxation techniques.

Medication to Alleviate Stress

All stress-reduction exercise techniques are preferable to the use of stress-reducing drugs, especially tranquilizers and mood-elevating drugs, which have addicting potential. But sometimes relaxation techniques fail. When this happens, your doctor may suggest you try a particular medication to mitigate the effects of stress on your body. A word about some of them.

Beta blockers interfere with the effects of adrenaline by blunting increases in heart rate and blood pressure. These drugs have been effective in decreasing such manifestations of anxiety as tremors and palpitations. They have also been given to addicts during the withdrawal period.

However, sudden termination of beta blocker therapy can, itself, cause withdrawal symptoms, including anxiety, shaking, sweating, and rapid heart rate. In patients with coronary heart disease, angina can be aggravated when beta blockers are abruptly stopped.

Side effects of beta-blocking drugs include very low heart rates and blood pressure, asthma attacks, and mental depression. They can also interfere with the control of diabetes and tend to raise cholesterol levels.

Minor tranquilizers, such as Valium, are commonly used in the treatment of anxiety disorders. But their use can result in major addictions. Withdrawal can be life-threatening. Some patients have a paradoxical reaction to these drugs, becoming aroused instead of relaxed. Fortunately, these drugs do not interact with the most commonly prescribed blood pressure and diabetes medications.

Tricyclic antidepressants such as amitriptyline (Elavil) have significant cardiac side effects. Like all these other drugs, they should be taken only under the supervision of a physician.

William Harvey observed 350 years ago that "every affection of the mind that is attended with either pain or pleasure, hope or fear, is the cause of an agitation whose influence extends to the heart." Emotional stress plays a major role in coronary heart disease. Stress reduction techniques can decrease cholesterol levels, reduce high blood pressure, and retard atherosclerosis.

Only you will know whether you're really practicing stress reduction, the same way that you alone know if you're exercising and following your particular level of the Nutrition Plan. Oh, your husband or wife probably suspects if you're not. But you're definitely the only one who can dedicate yourself to improve, to bring your stress score toward zero.

2 *Three-Month Evaluation*

Here we are at a major evaluation point for the class, as it will be for you—three months into the program. As you found out from Nick at Checkpoint 1, we lost one member of the original orientation group: Ed Donaldson. How were our remaining four friends doing on their countdowns toward zero?

MARIE CORELLI, despite the help of the Basic Heart Maintenance diet, followed by the Advanced Heart Repair diet and greatly increased fiber, along with a more regular schedule of exercise, had not lowered her LDL from the last value of 190. Her HDL was the same, 40, which might have been due to her continued inability to cut her smoking from two packs a day.

But Marie admitted she needed help and tried nicotine gum. She began exercising harder and more consistently, and her exercise score dropped to about 1½ as she began swimming more laps in the hope of reaching 1. All in all, she was starting to feel less like she was dying and more like she had a chance at life, despite the frustrating fact that her total score was still high risk. She gave herself a new stress score of 2, down from 2⅔.

I added a first-line drug, cholestyramine, to her regimen in the hope of driving down her LDL.

Marie's Score:

$$\left[\frac{LDL}{10} - \frac{HDL}{5}\right] + 2\left[\begin{array}{c}\# \text{ OF PACKS} \\ \text{PER DAY}\end{array}\right] + \begin{array}{c}\text{EXERCISE} \\ \text{SCORE}\end{array} + \begin{array}{c}\text{STRESS} \\ \text{SCORE}\end{array} + \frac{SBP - 130}{20} = \underline{\quad}$$

$$[\ 19\ -\ 8\ ] + \quad 4 \quad + \quad 1\tfrac{1}{2} \quad + \quad 2 \quad + \quad 0 \quad = 18\tfrac{1}{2}$$

CARLA PETERS was justifiably proud of herself. She'd lost 30 pounds in three months, lowered her initial LDL of 196 to 132, raised her HDL from 40 to an excellent 52, improved her six-week score of 2 for exercise down to 1, and felt so euphoric she attained a score of only ⅓ for stress. Her blood pressure was normal. From a starting total score that was high risk, she'd made it to the low-risk range.

She told Nick she wanted to try the stricter Advanced Heart Repair diet. He agreed, in order to try to drive her LDL down closer to 100, and added psyllium as supplemental fiber.

Carla's Score:

$$\left[\frac{LDL}{10} - \frac{HDL}{5}\right] + 2\left[\begin{array}{c}\# \text{ OF PACKS} \\ \text{PER DAY}\end{array}\right] + \begin{array}{c}\text{EXERCISE} \\ \text{SCORE}\end{array} + \begin{array}{c}\text{STRESS} \\ \text{SCORE}\end{array} + \frac{SBP - 130}{20} = \underline{\quad}$$

$$[\ 13\ -\ 10\ ] + \quad 0 \quad + \quad 1 \quad + \quad \tfrac{1}{3} \quad + \quad 0 \quad = 4\tfrac{1}{3}$$

FRANK KELSEY continued to lower his LDL. Initially 170, it was now 115. He accomplished this through diet, exercise, and reducing stress. His HDL inched up from 50 to 56, exercise was now 1, and his stress score remained 0, for he was no longer impotent and no longer worried about his health. His blood pressure remained 0 as well. He was now in the low-risk range.

In at attempt to get his LDL all the way down to 100, Nick prescribed an aggressive increase in his natural fiber intake, in the form of daily oat bran.

Frank's Score:

$$\left[\frac{LDL}{10} - \frac{HDL}{5}\right] + 2\left[\begin{array}{c}\text{\# OF PACKS}\\\text{PER DAY}\end{array}\right] + \begin{array}{c}\text{EXERCISE}\\\text{SCORE}\end{array} + \begin{array}{c}\text{STRESS}\\\text{SCORE}\end{array} + \frac{SBP - 130}{20} = \underline{\quad}$$

$$[\ 12\ -\ 11\ ] +\qquad 0\qquad +\quad 1\quad +\quad 0\quad +\qquad 0\qquad = 2$$

TONY SPAGNOLA brought his LDL from the initial 111 down to 100, and his HDL from 25 up to 30. He completely stopped smoking, doing it slowly, and told me he was sure he would never smoke again. His exercise score held steady at 1. When he stopped worrying about the successfully completed construction project, his stress score went to 0. He was right on the borderline between medium and low risk.

I started him on Niacin to try to raise his HDL, since stopping smoking had not had sufficient effect by itself. Neither had exercise, and he was already at his ideal weight. It was possible his low HDL was hereditary and needed the help of a drug regimen to bring it to a cardioprotective level nearer 50.

Tony's Score:

$$\left[\frac{LDL}{10} - \frac{HDL}{5}\right] + 2\left[\begin{array}{c}\text{\# OF PACKS}\\\text{PER DAY}\end{array}\right] + \begin{array}{c}\text{EXERCISE}\\\text{SCORE}\end{array} + \begin{array}{c}\text{STRESS}\\\text{SCORE}\end{array} + \frac{SBP - 130}{20} = \underline{\quad}$$

$$[\ 10\ -\ 6\ ] +\qquad 0\qquad +\quad 1\quad +\quad 0\quad +\qquad 0\qquad = 5$$

6 Quit Smoking and Live!

It's important to speak the language, and I don't mean only medical terminology like hyperlipidemia or cardiac catheterization. Nick and I know how vital it is to maintain open lines of communication—two-way, of course—with South Philadelphia, with the CVI staff, and with our patients.

We do everything we can think of to keep these lines open, from one-on-one meetings to the newsletters periodically given out in the office and mailed to all CVI patients. In addition, Nick does a radio show every morning on WPEN and a monthly cable TV show.

We've both lectured enough to know it's an uphill battle to convince people—especially those who still feel fine—to alter their diet, lower their blood pressure, exercise, reduce stress, and stop smoking. But we keep trying, because education is vitally important if we are to stop the enormous death toll from heart disease.

Did you know that smokers who quit reduce their risk of a heart attack in less than one year? And that after two to three years, their risk is about the same as that of someone who never smoked? So it should be amply obvious what needs to be done, and easy to do it. Right?

Wrong. What we hear most often in relation to smoking is a flat denial that it's an addiction; yet most of our patients admit that they just don't know why they can't stop puffing.

It has been more than twenty-five years since the Surgeon General earmarked cigarette smoking as the single most important preventable cause of death in the United States. By now, most Americans know that those warning labels on packs of cigarettes are not offering up the latest horoscopes. Smoking is not just a bad habit, so if you've been unable to stop, there's a reason for your failure. Smoking is a *proven addiction*. This is why 30 percent of adult Americans continue to smoke, despite overwhelming evidence they're killing themselves.

At CVI, we have two forms for our smokers to fill out. The first is a rating scale for smokers: The higher your score, the more dependent you probably are on smoking. The second is a questionnaire to help us determine how confident you are about being able to quit: This time, the higher your score, the better, because if you've answered honestly, you should have sufficient confidence to resist smoking in most difficult situations.

If you are a smoker, we've included copies of both forms at the end of this chapter (see pp. 166–67). And if you smoke, it's time you stop fooling yourself. Don't rationalize about your addiction. Don't pretend you're not seriously endangering your health. You must bring your smoking risk factor score down to zero.

The effects of smoking read like a list of the plagues: CHD, lung cancer, obstructive lung disease, stroke, peripheral vascular disease, abdominal aneurysms, peptic ulcer disease, and cancers of the oral cavity, larynx, esophagus, and bladder. The list alone should scare you half to death. Of the 550,000 people who die of coronary disease every year, 30 to 40 percent can probably blame cigarette smoking. If you smoke, your chances of dying of coronary disease are twice as high as that of nonsmokers. The more you smoke, the higher your risk, and the number of cigarettes you smoke each day is more critical than the number of years spent smoking.

The disastrous consequences of cigarette smoking are especially evident when other risk factors are also present. And if you've been counting on your filter tips to save you, forget it. They offer no protection whatsoever.

If you are a smoker, it's also way past time you gave serious consideration to the people around you. Passive exposure to your cigarette smoke increases coronary risk for everyone forced to breathe the same air. If the welfare of strangers doesn't concern you, the health of your loved ones certainly should. This means not just quitting yourself, but creating a smoke-free environment at home and at work. Toward this end, there is a strong regulatory move to eliminate smoking entirely from public places. You would have to be remarkably self-absorbed not to notice that smoking has become socially unacceptable.

But the ads still run. The stereotype of the male smoker broadened, in the course of about twenty years, from the Marlboro Man to the teenager lounging against a street pole, trying to look cool. Today, things have changed again, predictably not for the better. Have you noticed how many advertisements are now aimed at the approximately 25 million American women who smoke cigarettes? This represents a decrease since 1965, but those women who smoke are likely to smoke more heavily today than they did in the past, and smoking risk increases with the number of cigarettes smoked a day. Teen-age girls are beginning to smoke at a younger age—more girls than boys smoke between the ages of seventeen and nineteen.

Women who smoke are two to six times more likely to suffer a heart attack than nonsmoking women, depending on how many cigarettes they smoke. A woman who smokes very heavily may have her risk approach that of a man. Heavy smokers tend to have earlier menopause, also increasing risk.

Those who smoke and take birth control pills have a very high risk of heart disease, being thirty-nine times more likely to have a heart attack, and up to twenty-two times more likely to have a stroke, than women who neither smoke nor use birth control pills.

Remarkable that anyone actually continues to smoke, isn't it?

These were the facts presented to the orientation class. Of the nine remaining class members, Marie was the heaviest smoker. She was finding it very difficult to stop, and told me about it:

"Don't you see, I can't do it, Dr. Dowinsky. It's too much. I've been putting it all on James [her husband], for smoking in front of me. But even when he's not home, I feel like I'll go crazy if I don't have a cigarette. I just keep looking at my cigarettes. And the urge to take one and light it up drives me nuts!"

Marie has to find the courage to quit and the inner motivation to carry through on it. Of all ex-smokers, 90 percent finally stop without special treatments or programs—self-motivation. Marie already has coronary heart disease. And smoking accelerates heart disease by its direct effects on the lining of the artery, as well as by increasing LDL and triglycerides, lowering HDL, and causing the blood to clot more easily and quickly. An acute heart attack represents a rude awakening for most patients, as it did for Marie.

Fortunately, it's never too late to stop smoking.

What Happens When Smoke Gets in Your Heart?

Nicotine and carbon monoxide are the two components of cigarette smoke that have been most incriminated in the development of coronary heart disease. Nicotine, the addictive component, stimulates the release of adrenaline to increase heart rate and blood pressure. It also activates the nervous system to produce a state of arousal. Blood vessels under the skin constrict, redirecting blood flow to the muscles. All these effects combine to increase the workload of the heart.

Simultaneously, carbon monoxide (CO) attaches itself to red blood cells, dislodging oxygen molecules. This reduces the availability of oxygen carried to the heart muscle by each red blood cell.

If the coronary arteries are partially blocked, the nicotine-stimulated increased oxygen demand, combined with a CO-induced decreased oxygen supply, can trigger an angina attack.

Cigarette smoke also causes a decrease in the diameter of the coronary arteries. Add to the problem of narrowed coronary arteries the fact that the blood of smokers coagulates more easily than that of nonsmokers. The decreased diameter of the coronary arteries and increased tendency toward clot formation probably account for the link between smoking and sudden death as well as heart attack.

Furthermore, nicotine and carbon monoxide make the heart more prone to rhythm disturbances. And finally, smokers have difficulty elevating their low levels of HDL even while exercising.

Easier Said Than Done

But nicotine is one of the most addictive substances known to humankind. It is six to eight times more addictive than alcohol. Like alcohol, heroin, and cocaine, it can produce both physical and psychological dependence. Withdrawal symptoms are very real—so real that the relapse rate among smokers who attempt to quit is as high as 70 percent after three months without a cigarette.

But I'm telling you, there's no alternative. Yes, it can be hard, very hard, but the known benefits of quitting are an increased life expectancy, an improved lung capacity, a reduced risk of heart attack, lowered blood pressure, a diminished smoker's cough, and an enhanced sense of smell and taste.

Quit and live!

If you really want to quit, you, like Marie, must arrive at

some inner form of motivation. Other people, doctors included, can't substitute for your own will. Scare tactics are pointless. They only cause anxiety and aggravate the problem. Putting you under too much stress can actually lead to an increase in smoking.

In the past few years, smoking cessation programs have proliferated. Some advise patients to reduce by 10 to 20 percent the number of cigarettes smoked each day before even attempting to quit completely. Others recommend switching to brands lower in tar and nicotine before quitting. Techniques involving rapid smoking, trapping smoke in the mouth while concentrating on unpleasant thoughts, hypnosis, and acupuncture all have variable results; unfortunately, the one-year success rates for all these programs range only from 10 to 40 percent.

But whatever method you choose, *you must stop smoking.* Knowing how hard quitting can be, it is essential for your doctor to take an active role in helping you. It's usually that much harder without support, when a smoker tries to quit alone. For one thing, it is crucial to recognize the withdrawal symptoms and know they're temporary. The active involvement of your doctor can improve your motivation, and he/she can provide treatment of withdrawal symptoms as they occur.

The smoking cessation program we use was modified from a study conducted by Dr. C. Barr Taylor of the Stanford University School of Medicine. It has achieved very good results.

ELEVEN-STEP SMOKING CESSATION PROGRAM

Step 1—Get the Message!

There are no alternatives. You simply must quit. Your doctor should be the one to make you understand that this is not a negotiable issue.

Step 2—*Are You Willing to Quit?*

Most smokers want to quit. But if you have no desire to quit despite having been told about the hazardous effects of smoking, setting a future date with your doctor to discuss the issue once again seems the best bet.

Step 3—*Select the Best Technique*

The Rating Scale for Smokers at the end of this chapter (p. 166) will help you determine your degree of smoking dependency. If your score shows you to be highly dependent, it's unlikely you can quit on your own, and you may even need drug intervention and more intensive group support.

Step 4—*Ask Your Doctor to Educate You About Withdrawal*

You must know what to expect after that last cigarette. You may need nicotine replacement therapy (nicotine gum or the new nicotine patch) to blunt withdrawal symptoms. Such aids will relieve the effects of nicotine withdrawal while you get through the first critical seven- to ten-day period, and I'll tell you more about them shortly. Be assured that most withdrawal symptoms occur in short bursts, generally lasting only a few minutes and gradually decreasing in intensity. They include restlessness, irritability, and anxiety. Drowsiness may also occur. You may awaken from sleep or show marked impatience, confusion, and impaired concentration. Your appetite will probably increase, usually leading to weight gain, though this may not occur if you're following a diet. There will be strong cravings for a cigarette.

Most withdrawal symptoms reach their maximum intensity twenty-four to forty-eight hours after the last cigarette, and gradually diminish over a ten-day period. But the desire to smoke, especially under stress, can persist for months or even years.

Most patients who fail to get through this period do so because they don't know what to expect and become frightened. Apprehension often leads to lighting up a cigarette, which unfortunately quickly alleviates the withdrawal symptoms. Just remember, regular exercise, deep breathing exercises, and substitute outlets for relaxation will ultimately create a far greater sense of well-being than you now feel by smoking.

Step 5—Set a Quitting Date

Agreeing with your doctor on a quitting date is one of the most important aspects of any cessation program. Some doctors have their patients sign a contract committing to a specific deadline. This formalizes the process.

Step 6—Preparatory Measures

Keep a diary. Go through self-education materials. Try to eliminate situations in which you usually smoke before the quitting date is reached. This makes stopping easier on the date. You'll be amazed how much your diary discloses, especially with respect to your specific reasons for smoking.

Step 7—Coping with the Urge to Smoke

How great is your confidence in your ability to resist the urge to smoke? Try the Confidence Questionnaire for Smokers at the end of this chapter (p. 167). If your score is above 35, you should do well. A score of 1 or 2 for a given area may signal the need for more help. If your score is under 35, you may need nicotine replacement therapy.

Step 8—Involving Family and Friends

Your family should be educated to provide support. Friends can also help. If family members and friends are smokers, it will certainly be best if they refrain from smoking in your presence. This will be less important after seven to ten days when withdrawal symptoms are no longer as prominent. If your confidence score is very high, you may be better able to tolerate other smokers.

Step 9—Additional Aids

Relapses occur when patients drink alcohol, especially those with low confidence scores. They frequently have a prior history of alcohol abuse. If you have such a problem, you'll need appropriate alcohol rehabilitation counseling.

Exercise can relieve stress and provide an outlet for frustrations. It also helps reduce the weight gain that usually follows abstinence. Stress reduction techniques will provide additional support.

Step 10—Follow-Up Care

A call to your doctor, or an office visit, can spot problems and reinforce confidence. Filling out the Confidence Questionnaire again can identify specific areas that need further work. Once you've gotten through the first six months, follow-up phone calls should be made by your doctor every six months to check for any relapse.

Step 11—Ex-Smokers' Clinics

If you have been able to stop smoking for at least six months, you may want to spend time helping others to achieve this goal. Group counseling sessions can bring together smokers who are attempting to quit with those who have already been successful.

Nicotine Replacement Therapy

Nicotine gum: Nicotine chewing gum (Nicorette) is available by prescription and can be an effective aid in smoking cessation programs. Each stick of gum contains 2 mg of nicotine. Gum containing 4 mg has been marketed in Canada and Europe and has proved effective with heavy smokers.

The gum not only provides a noninhaled form of nicotine but also acts as an oral replacement for the cigarette. It is usually effective only when the chewing gum, a formal smoking cessation program, and behavior modification are all combined to break the addiction.

Be aware that chewing nicotine gum can shift the addiction to the gum. It's advisable to get off the nicotine gum within four months. The gum should be chewed very slowly, just enough to produce mild tingling in your mouth. Surprisingly, it is not always made clear that smoking must stop *before* you start using the gum.

Obviously, because of nicotine's cardiac effects, patients who have had a recent heart attack, unstable angina, or seriously irregular heart rhythm should be advised against using the nicotine gum. But it is safer than smoking, for it does not contain carbon monoxide, tars, and other toxins present in inhaled smoke.

Nicotine patch: Nicotine-releasing adhesive patches have been recently approved by the U.S. Food and Drug Administration. They reduce the craving to smoke, thereby easing withdrawal symptoms, while preventing a high level of nicotine from developing rapidly. But this is very important. You must stop smoking before the patch is applied. Heart attacks have been reported in some patients who continued smoking while wearing the patch.

A Final Word on Smoking

The tobacco industry has promoted the impression that low-yield brands of cigarettes are safer than others. Some recent advertising campaigns for these brands have been directed specifically toward women. But these low-yield cigarettes do not protect against heart attacks. Abstinence remains the only preventive measure, if you are to bring your smoking risk factor score to zero. And you *must* bring it to zero.

The rating scale and questionnaire follow. If you're a smoker, use them as a guide to your smoking habits.

RATING SCALE FOR SMOKERS

This modified Horn-Russell rating scale is used to measure your degree of dependence on nicotine. There are 11 questions. Each is scored 0–3 points. A maximum of 33 points (3 points × 11 questions) can be obtained. The scale is as follows:

> 3 = almost always
> 2 = usually
> 1 = occasionally
> 0 = never

(a) It is easy to talk and get along with other people when I am smoking.
(b) I feel more confident when smoking with other people.
(c) Handling a cigarette is part of the enjoyment of smoking.
(d) Smoking helps me think and concentrate.
(e) When I run out of cigarettes I find it unbearable until I can get them again.
(f) I smoke more often when I am worried or angry about something.
(g) One reason I smoke is it tastes so good.
(h) Smoking cheers me up.
(i) Smoking helps me to get going when I am tired.
(j) Smoking helps me while I am busy and working hard and I enjoy smoking at that time.
(k) I am very much aware of the fact when I am not smoking.

SOURCE: Modified from M. A. Russell, J. Peto, and U. A. Patel, "The Classification of Smoking by Factorial Structure of Motives." *Journal of the Royal Statistical Society* (America). 137:313–64, 1974.

CONFIDENCE QUESTIONNAIRE FOR SMOKERS

This questionnaire rates your ability to resist cigarette smoking for each listed situation. Please enter a number from 1 to 5, based on the following scale, for each item:

5 points = very confident
4 points = fairly confident
3 points = possibly confident
2 points = slightly confident
1 point = not confident

ITEM	CONFIDENCE SCORE
1. When you feel impatient	_____
2. When you want to relax	_____
3. When you want to concentrate	_____
4. When someone offers you a cigarette	_____
5. When someone around you is smoking or has a pack of cigarettes visible	_____
6. When you feel worried, upset, tense, or anxious about a certain situation	_____
7. After eating a meal	_____
8. When you feel fatigued and need a lift	_____
9. When you want to improve your self-image or self-esteem	_____
10. When you are out drinking alcoholic beverages	_____

SOURCE: Modified from M. M. Condiotte and E. Lichtenstein, "Self-Efficacy and Relapse in Smoking Cessation Programs." *Journal of Consulting and Clinical Psychology.* 49(5):648–58, October 1981.

7 And If All Else Fails . . .

Some of our patients find that they've still failed to achieve their cholesterol goals—usually after spending a minimum of three months progressing through the Philadelphia Formula Nutrition Plan. At this point, Nick and I will normally start drug therapy to help bring the cholesterol risk factor score down toward zero. Marie was in this category.

All the drugs discussed in this chapter must be taken under a doctor's supervision. The primary focus is on drug treatment for elevated total and LDL cholesterol. Secondary is the problem of HDL under 35 mg/dl, in conjunction with high total and LDL cholesterol levels.

If you were not updating your cholesterol numbers every six weeks in order to monitor your progress, once drug therapy is initiated, you will need to have your LDL and total cholesterol levels measured at four- to six-week intervals. If, after three months, the drug therapy is working and is to be continued, you will need to be seen at least every four months. If your response to the drug is not adequate, and additional or different drugs are required, it will be necessary to have more frequent check-ups to monitor possible side effects.

As a participant in the Philadelphia Formula Countdown toward zero, you and your doctor monitor these factors closely, at regular intervals, for your own complete safety and peace of mind.

FIRST-LINE THERAPY: BILE-ACID SEQUESTRANTS

Bile-acid sequestrants (cholestyramine and colestipol) have been shown to lower LDL by 15 to 30 percent. Additionally, both have long-term safety records and the added benefit of raising HDL. They are good choices for the young, and for safety-conscious individuals, but may not be the right choice for the elderly, who tend to become constipated more easily and to have more gastrointestinal problems than younger people. These drugs may also not be the best choice for those with hemorrhoids, recurrent symptoms of peptic ulcer disease, or hiatal hernia.

A drawback of both cholestyramine and colestipol is their tendency to elevate triglyceride levels. But for patients whose triglycerides are normal, the bile-acid sequestrants are the initial mainstay of cholesterol-lowering therapy.

They are extremely safe because they are not absorbed. They function by promoting cholesterol removal from the bloodstream by the liver for bile-acid (cholesterol) synthesis, and by binding the bile acids in the intestine, causing cholesterol loss through the stools. The dose must be taken with a major meal to maximize this binding in the intestines.

Cholestyramine (Questran) and colestipol (Colestid) are both granular powders to be mixed in a liquid. They're available in individual packets or in a bulk (scoop) package, and a flavored cholestyramine candy bar has recently been marketed. It is far less expensive to purchase the bulk than the smaller packages.

If you find yourself suffering from constipation and other

gastrointestinal problems, psyllium will help alleviate these effects. A nonabsorbable stool softener, or dried apricots or prunes, will help you avoid constipation.

The bile sequestrants may be taken for a lifetime. They are not toxic and, because they're not absorbed into the bloodstream, have no effect on the blood or organs. However, they may interfere with the absorption of fat-soluble vitamins or common drugs such as digoxin, thiazides, or warfarin (Coumadin), making it vital that your primary physician is always kept up to date on all medications you are taking.

SECOND-LINE THERAPY

Nicotinic acid (Niacin) is a good choice where cost is a major concern. The most economical drug available, it's a water-soluble B vitamin (B_3) that both lowers serum cholesterol and raises HDL.

Niacin decreases the liver's production of VLDL (very low-density lipoprotein cholesterol) by 75 percent, and cuts down LDL cholesterol by about 25 percent. Good HDL cholesterol rises by 20 to 40 percent.

Niacin can be purchased in health stores without a prescription, but like the other cholesterol-lowering drugs described here, you should use it only under a doctor's supervision. There may be side effects.

For example, in one of his recent studies, Nick found that long-term use of Niacin can have a toxic effect on the liver. And there are other, less threatening side effects.

Some women, both during and after menopause, experience flushing when taking Niacin. It can cause flushing in both men and women at all ages. If this is a problem, you can take aspirin half an hour before the Niacin. Itching is another possible side effect. It can be minimized by trying sustained-release preparations only after meals.

Blood testing will be necessary to monitor liver function, blood sugar, and uric-acid levels. Niacin is relatively safe *under a doctor's supervision,* and may also be used in conjunction with a bile-acid sequestrant. It should certainly be considered when cholestyramine or colestipol are contraindicated. In cases where triglycerides are elevated along with total cholesterol, Niacin is the drug of choice.

It should not be used if there is any history of active ulcer disease, liver disease, gout, gastritis, high uric acid, poorly controlled diabetes, or significant irregularity of the heartbeat.

Dosages vary from 50 mg taken three times a day, to 1 gram taken three times a day.

THIRD-LINE THERAPY

Gemfibrozil (Lopid) is a fibric-acid derivative, effective in lowering LDL cholesterol by 10 to 20 percent and triglycerides by up to 50 percent. Ten to 20 percent increases in HDL cholesterol can occur. Usually well tolerated, the most common side effects are gastrointestinal. Lopid may predispose patients to the development of gallstones. Blood tests and liver tests must be done repeatedly.

Probucol (Lorelco) is another third-line drug that can lower LDL by about 10 percent, but it can also lower HDL by about 20 percent. Unlike Questran and Colestid, Niacin and Lopid, Lorelco has not yet been shown to reduce coronary risk in humans, but a large Swedish study is now under way to test its ability to promote reversal of atherosclerosis.

Side effects include gastrointestinal problems, which may be followed by electrocardiogram abnormalities. This drug has been used in combination therapy for patients with resistant high cholesterol.

Another third-line drug is lovastatin (Mevacor), the drug to which Nick compared Niacin in his study, in order to deter-

172   *The Heart Repair Manual*

mine relative liver toxicity. Mevacor has only been available for a few years, but is expected to show significant reduction in mortality on long-term follow-up studies. It is well tolerated by the elderly.

Lovastatin is an excellent choice for patients receiving multiple medications, who have extensive disease or very severe forms of high cholesterol. It is the most powerful drug currently available for reducing serum cholesterol, quickly producing sizable decreases. It also raises HDL.

Lovastatin is very specific in inhibiting the most important enzyme used by the liver to manufacture cholesterol. It can produce up to 45 percent reductions in LDL by increasing the number of LDL receptors on the liver, thus increasing LDL removal from the blood. It also lowers triglycerides. It is very effective for those with hereditary high cholesterol, and can raise HDL by approximately 10 percent.

Of major concern is the fact that long-term use of such drugs may elevate liver function enzymes. In Nick's study, Mevacor appeared to have less effect on the liver than Niacin. Regardless, during the first fifteen months of taking Mevacor, you must have your blood tested monthly to monitor your liver function, and after fifteen months, at set periods determined by your doctor.

Lovastatin is the most effective drug now available for lowering cholesterol. More follow-up studies are needed to determine its long-term safety and its effect on reducing the incidence of heart attack and cardiac deaths. This data is almost surely forthcoming and should support long-term use.

Very recently, two new lovastatin-like drugs—pravastatin (Pravachol) and simvastatin (Zocor)—were approved by the Food and Drug Administration for the treatment of hypercholesterolemia. They are expected to be of comparable effectiveness.

THE ADDITIONAL PROBLEM OF RAISING HDL CHOLESTEROL

As you know, a separate but related problem often arises when total cholesterol is elevated and HDL is low (under 35 mg/dl). Most therapy is primarily aimed at reducing LDL and total cholesterol, but it's very important to raise your HDL as well. Questran, Colestid, and Niacin will all accomplish this to varying degrees. Niacin is often preferable because of its greater ability to elevate HDL while lowering total serum cholesterol. Lopid and Mevacor also raise HDL.

Tables 10A and 10B list the medications routinely used to treat dyslipidemias (abnormal concentrations of LDL, VLDL, or HDL).

COMBINATION THERAPY

Occasionally, there may not be an adequate cholesterol-lowering response to a single drug. In this situation, your doctor may want to consider combination therapy.

One useful combination, especially for those with normal triglycerides but elevated cholesterol, is Questran or Colestid along with either Niacin or Mevacor. The bile-acid sequestrant combined with Mevacor can decrease LDL cholesterol by 50 to 60 percent. The sequestrant combined with Niacin raises HDL.

In conclusion, your doctor, you, and your family, all working together, can markedly improve the chances for success with drug therapy. Your doctor must of course provide you with regular feedback on your cholesterol levels so that you know whether the current treatment is a success or a failure. If a specific treatment is unsuccessful, it can then be promptly altered. Follow-up appointments should be scheduled at regular intervals, because close supervision is very important.

Above all, never lose heart. As long as you never stop trying, you will ultimately move your risk factors closer to zero.

Table 10A

Medications Routinely Used to Treat Dyslipidemias

	Drug	Reduce CHD Risk?	Long-Term Safety?
First-Line Therapy	Cholestyramine (Questran)	Yes (LRC-CPPT)	Yes
	Colestipol (Colestid)	Yes (CLAS)	Yes
Second-Line Therapy	Nicotinic acid (Niacin)	Yes (CDP)	Yes
Third-Line Therapy	Gemfibrozil (Lopid)	Yes (Helsinki)	Yes
	Probucol (Lorelco)	Not Yet Known	Not Available
	Lovastatin (Mevacor)	Not Yet Known	Not Available

NOTE: References to studies or groups doing the studies: LRC-CPPT = Lipid Research Clinics: Cholesterol Primary Prevention Trial; CLAS = Cholesterol-Lowering Atherosclerosis Study; CDP = Coronary Drug Project; Helsinki = Helsinki Heart Study.

Table 10B
Medications—Be Aware of/Test; Adverse Effects

Drug	Be Aware of/Test	Adverse Effects
Cholestyramine	Dosing of other medications	Constipation, bloating, fullness
Colestipol	Dosing of other medications	Constipation, bloating, fullness
Nicotinic acid	Uric acid, glucose (sugar), liver tests	Flushing, itching, gout, high uric acid, high sugar, hepatitis
Gemfibrozil	Blood count, liver tests	Gastrointestinal symptoms, muscle aches, possible increase in gallstones
Probucol	ECG, HDL values	Diarrhea, abdominal pain, abnormal ECG change
Lovastatin	Liver tests, muscle enzyme test, eye examinations	Hepatitis (2%), muscle aches, skin rash, headaches

Conclusion

The people of South Philadelphia retain the old tradition of warmth toward their physicians. There is a huge geriatric population, and the older patients and their families extend the intense loyalty they feel for each other to those who take care of them.

The result is that in the neighborhoods around CVI, doctors are treated with great respect. Families offer their thanks to their doctor, and this doesn't change in times of turmoil, of long hospitalizations, or even with the death of a loved one.

I guess you realize by now that Steve and I are passionate about seeing that there are fewer and fewer deaths.

How did the four remaining members of the orientation group, whose progress we're following, do at the nine-month checkpoint? Let's take a look, one last time, to see if any of them have reached zero.

MARIE CORELLI grew happier and more confident with every week that passed. By the end of nine months, she'd succeeded in lowering her LDL to 106, but she needed lovastatin (Mevacor) to accomplish this. Her HDL was finally up to 48. The nicotine gum didn't help her at all, but the patch did, and she actually stopped smoking, though she was still experiencing periods of intense craving for a cigarette. So far, she'd overcome them, one by one.

For exercise, she made it down to 1. The state of her health and finances were no longer of such overwhelming importance. She no longer viewed life with pessimism and dread. Her stress score finally zeroed out, and her husband and daughter told her they hadn't seen her so relaxed in a very long time.

Her high-risk score, originally 22%, at nine months was now so low risk as to be almost counted down to zero:

$$\left[\frac{LDL}{10} - \frac{HDL}{5}\right] + 2\left[\begin{array}{c}\#\ OF\ PACKS\\ PER\ DAY\end{array}\right] + \begin{array}{c}EXERCISE\\SCORE\end{array} + \begin{array}{c}STRESS\\SCORE\end{array} + \frac{SBP - 130}{20} = \underline{\quad}$$

$$[\ 11\ -\ 10\ ] +\quad 0\quad +\quad 1\quad +\quad 0\quad +\quad 0\quad = 2$$

CARLA PETERS in every way astonished herself. At nine months, she'd not only maintained her weight loss but was slowly and steadily losing even more, about ½ pound a week.

Her blood pressure was normal, her mild diabetes less of a risk since she was dieting and exercising aerobically.

Carla had gained so much confidence, she'd gone back to teaching. She even started seeing one of the other teachers in her school, and by the time of this check-in, it looked like it might be getting serious. Her LDL was down to 110, her HDL was 60. Exercise was down to 0 and so was stress. She was praised by Steve and me, and by her classmates, for her exceptional success.

Carla's starting score was in the high-risk range, at 18. At nine months, her winning score was:

$$\left[\frac{LDL}{10} - \frac{HDL}{5}\right] + 2\left[\substack{\text{\# OF PACKS} \\ \text{PER DAY}}\right] + \substack{\text{EXERCISE} \\ \text{SCORE}} + \substack{\text{STRESS} \\ \text{SCORE}} + \frac{SBP - 130}{20} = \underline{\quad}$$

$$[\ 11\ -\ 12\ ] +\qquad 0\qquad +\quad 0\quad +\quad 0\quad +\qquad 0\qquad = 0$$

FRANK KELSEY's LDL was down to 112, his HDL was still 56. Exercise was still 1, stress 0, blood pressure normal. From an initial moderately high risk score of 14, he now had an almost perfect score:

$$\left[\frac{LDL}{10} - \frac{HDL}{5}\right] + 2\left[\substack{\text{\# OF PACKS} \\ \text{PER DAY}}\right] + \substack{\text{EXERCISE} \\ \text{SCORE}} + \substack{\text{STRESS} \\ \text{SCORE}} + \frac{SBP - 130}{20} = \underline{\quad}$$

$$[\ 11\ -\ 11\ ] +\qquad 0\qquad +\quad 1\quad +\quad 0\quad +\qquad 0\qquad = 1$$

TONY SPAGNOLA's LDL remained at 100: his HDL was up to 35. Smoking remained 0. Exercise was also 0, since he'd goaded his wife, Lou, into taking the other bike out of the garage and racing him on it, which made the time go faster and the distance that much easier. He still hadn't managed to beat her, even once, at the nine-month mark. Stress remained 0. His starting score had been just above medium risk at 10⅓. Now, it was a good low risk:

$$\left[\frac{LDL}{10} - \frac{HDL}{5}\right] + 2\left[\substack{\text{\# OF PACKS} \\ \text{PER DAY}}\right] + \substack{\text{EXERCISE} \\ \text{SCORE}} + \substack{\text{STRESS} \\ \text{SCORE}} + \frac{SBP - 130}{20} = \underline{\quad}$$

$$[\ 10\ -\ 7\ ] +\qquad 0\qquad +\quad 0\quad +\quad 0\quad +\qquad 0\qquad = 3$$

Your Own Progress

How will you be doing after nine months of the Philadelphia Formula program? If you've been filling in your risk factor scores, you'll easily be able to see how far you've already come. But the nine-month mark isn't an end point. As we discussed before, this is a program for life.

If you haven't yet started to follow the program, what in the world are you waiting for? Thousands of others before you have grabbed the gold ring for a healthier, more vibrant life. We stand here now, face to face with your turn to do just that.

Don't blow it! You've read through the entire *Heart Repair Manual,* and that was certainly the first vital step. But you can't benefit from the Philadelphia Formula by indefinitely sitting around thinking about it.

Your whole life's at stake here. Is that a big enough incentive? We sincerely hope it is: your life expectancy, your quality of life, every aspect of your existence. It's time to stop procrastinating, now. Time to admit you need to make some changes. Time to stop jeopardizing your life.

After all the time we've spent with you, you can't ask us to believe you won't even try. You can't expect us to have any doubts at all that you'll ultimately succeed in getting your risk factors to zero.

But you have to take this first major step. You have to get started. This program is not one of the many things in life you're forced to do that have no benefit for you. It's not one of those things that just don't feel right. You *know* our program is different. It felt right the minute you started reading this book. That's why you kept on reading.

The Philadelphia Formula Countdown program is a feel-good thing, like a steambath or a massage or a long-awaited vacation to a place you've always wanted to visit. Something that you yourself choose to do, that you have complete control over.

It's time now for renewal. To be invigorated. To hand yourself your best chance for a longer, happier, healthier life. To be very, very proud of yourself.

So come with us. Do it now. It's only hard while you're sitting around contemplating whether to do it or not. The first step is forming that alliance with your family doctor. Use his/her knowledge and concern for your continuing welfare. And us? Use our knowledge, too. Don't forget about Steve and me just because you've finished reading this book. We're not out of your life as long as we stay in touch.

Steve now has his own private practice, quite close to CVI, so those brain-storming sessions that produced the Philadelphia Formula program haven't ended, and we don't expect they're about to. They keep us both perpetually sharp. Do some brain-storming with us, by writing to us, care of W. W. Norton & Company, our publisher. Write to us whenever you need us. At the checkpoints. At the end of the nine months. In between. We want to hear from you. We want to know how your life's going. And ask your doctor to write, too.

Steve and I greatly value the time we've already spent together. Our partnership with our patients is one of the things that keeps us practicing with renewed zeal year after year. And now, we feel we're extending that partnership beyond Philadelphia—to you, to everyone who reads *The Heart Repair Manual.*

Please, give us your opinion of the program. How you feel about following it. Any suggestions you can make about how to improve it. Tell us how your life's going, now. How close you're getting to zero.

And, above all, don't let yourself down. It's up to you to end the war of attrition that could eventually choke the blood supply to your heart, your brain, your legs. The Philadelphia Formula arms you with the weapons you need to win the battle against coronary heart disease. Learning to use them requires self-discipline and motivation, but this should come easily, for it isn't a remote battle you're fighting for control of some foreign territory. It's a fight within your own body—for a healthier, longer, and more vigorous life. It is the closest possible encounter.

Appendices

A Fat and Cholesterol Comparison Composites

Let's take a look at the fat and cholesterol comparison tables that will help you choose food items relatively low in saturated fat. The information on total fat, percent calories from fat, and calories of each food item will be helpful if you're trying to lose weight.

When trying to lose weight, bear in mind that everyone's weight fluctuates from day to day. You may be faithful to your diet and yet, at your next weigh-in, find a gain rather than the expected loss in pounds.

Don't despair. This is perfectly normal. Simply stick to your diet, and the weight will start coming off again. Just never give up—on your diet or yourself.

Even if you don't need a weight-reducing diet, you know that you must modify the amount of cholesterol and saturated fat you eat. To do this, it will usually be sufficient to select items from the upper portion of each category on each list. But on Table 11, for example, the top item is kidneys, which are low in saturated fat but high in cholesterol. Just use your common sense.

You'll find yourself quickly internalizing these things. As we promised, you'll need to refer to the lists less and less often as you make the eating plan part of your way of life.

Table 11

Meats: Fat and Cholesterol Comparison Chart

Product (3½ oz, cooked)	Sat. Fat. (gm)	Chol. (mg)	Total Fat (gm)	% Calories from Fat	Total Calories
Beef					
Kidneys, simmered	1.1	387	3.4	21	144
Liver, braised	1.9	389	4.9	27	161
Round, top round, lean only, broiled	2.2	84	6.2	29	191
Round, top round, lean only, roasted	2.8	81	7.5	36	190
Round, full cut, lean only, choice, broiled	2.9	82	8.0	37	194
Round, bottom round, lean only, braised	3.4	96	9.7	39	222
Short loin, top loin, lean only, broiled	3.6	76	8.9	40	203
Wedge-bone sirloin, lean only, broiled	3.6	89	8.7	38	208
Short loin, tenderloin, lean only, broiled	3.6	84	9.3	41	204
Chuck, arm pot roast, lean only, braised	3.8	101	10.0	39	231
Short loin, T-bone steak, lean only, choice, broiled	4.2	80	10.4	44	214

Table 11 (*Continued*)

Product (3½ oz, cooked)	Sat. Fat. (gm)	Chol. (mg)	Total Fat (gm)	% Calories from Fat	Total Calories
Short loin, porterhouse steak, lean only, choice, broiled	4.3	80	10.8	45	218
Brisket, whole, lean only, braised	4.6	93	12.8	48	241
Rib eye, small end (ribs 10–12), lean only, choice, broiled	4.9	80	11.6	47	225
Rib, whole (ribs 6–12), lean only, roasted	5.8	81	13.8	52	240
Flank, lean only, choice, braised	5.9	71	13.8	51	244
Rib, large end (ribs 6–9), lean only, broiled	6.1	82	14.2	55	233
Chuck, blade roast, lean only, braised	6.2	106	15.3	51	270
Corned beef, cured brisket, cooked	6.3	98	19.0	68	251
Flank, lean and fat, choice, braised	6.6	72	15.5	54	257
Ground, lean, broiled medium	7.2	87	18.5	61	272
Round, full cut, lean and fat, choice, braised	7.3	84	18.2	60	274

Table 11 (*Continued*)

Product (3½ oz, cooked)	Sat. Fat. (gm)	Chol. (mg)	Total Fat (gm)	% Calories from Fat	Total Calories
Rib, short ribs, lean only, choice, braised	7.7	93	18.1	55	295
Salami, cured, cooked, smoked, 3–4 slices	9.0	65	20.7	71	262
Short loin, T-bone steak, lean and fat, choice, broiled	10.2	84	24.6	68	324
Chuck, arm pot roast, lean and fat, braised	10.7	99	26.0	67	350
Sausage, cured, cooked, smoked, about 2	11.4	67	26.9	78	312
Bologna, cured, 3–4 slices	12.1	58	28.5	82	312
Frankfurter, cured, about 2	12.0	61	28.5	82	315
Lamb					
Leg, lean only, roasted	3.0	89	8.2	39	191
Loin chop, lean only, broiled	4.1	94	9.4	39	215
Rib, lean only, roasted	5.7	88	12.3	48	232
Arm chop, lean only, braised	6.0	122	14.6	47	279
Rib, lean and fat, roasted	14.2	90	30.6	75	368

Table 11 (*Continued*)

Product (3½ oz, cooked)	Sat. Fat. (gm)	Chol. (mg)	Total Fat (gm)	% Calories from Fat	Total Calories
Pork					
Cured, ham steak, boneless, extra lean, unheated	1.4	45	4.2	31	122
Liver, braised	1.4	355	4.4	24	165
Kidneys, braised	1.5	480	4.7	28	151
Fresh, loin, tenderloin, lean only, roasted	1.7	93	4.8	26	166
Cured, shoulder, arm picnic, lean only, roasted	2.4	48	7.0	37	170
Cured, ham, boneless, regular, roasted	3.1	59	9.0	46	178
Fresh, leg (ham), shank half, lean only, roasted	3.6	92	10.5	44	215
Fresh, leg (ham), rump half, lean only, roasted	3.7	96	10.7	43	221
Fresh, loin, center loin, sirloin, lean only, roasted	4.5	91	13.1	49	240
Fresh, loin, sirloin, lean only, roasted	4.5	90	13.2	50	236

Table 11 (*Continued*)

Product (3½ oz, cooked)	Sat. Fat. (gm)	Chol. (mg)	Total Fat (gm)	% Calories from Fat	Total Calories
Fresh, loin, center rib, lean only roasted	4.8	79	13.8	51	245
Fresh, loin, top loin, lean only, roasted	4.8	79	13.8	51	245
Fresh, shoulder, blade, Boston, lean only, roasted	5.8	98	16.8	59	256
Fresh, loin, blade, lean only, roasted	6.6	89	19.3	62	279
Fresh, loin, sirloin, lean and fat, roasted	7.4	91	20.4	63	291
Cured, shoulder, arm picnic, lean and fat, roasted	7.7	58	21.4	69	280
Fresh, loin, center loin, lean and fat, roasted	7.9	91	21.8	64	305
Cured, shoulder, blade, roll, lean and fat, roasted	8.4	67	23.5	74	287
Fresh, Italian sausage, cooked	9.0	78	25.7	72	323
Fresh, bratwurst, cooked	9.3	60	25.9	77	301

Table 11 (*Continued*)

Product (3½ oz, cooked)	Sat. Fat. (gm)	Chol. (mg)	Total Fat (gm)	% Calories from Fat	Total Calories
Fresh, chitterlings, cooked	10.1	143	28.8	86	303
Cured, liver sausage, liverwurst	10.6	158	28.5	79	326
Cured, smoked link sausage, grilled	11.3	68	31.8	74	389
Fresh, spareribs, lean and fat, braised	11.8	121	30.3	69	397
Cured, salami, dry or hard	11.9	——	33.7	75	407
Bacon, fried	17.4	85	49.2	78	576
Veal					
Rump, lean only, roasted	——	128	2.2	13	156
Sirloin, lean only, roasted	——	128	3.2	19	153
Arm steak, lean only, cooked	——	90	5.3	24	200
Loin chop, lean only, cooked	——	90	6.7	29	207
Blade, lean only, cooked	——	90	7.8	33	211
Cutlet, medium fat, braised or broiled	4.8	128	11.0	37	271
Foreshank, medium fat, stewed	——	90	10.4	43	216
Plate, medium fat, stewed	——	90	21.2	63	303
Rib, medium fat, roasted	7.1	128	16.9	70	218

Table 11 (*Continued*)

Product (3½ oz, cooked)	Sat. Fat. (gm)	Chol. (mg)	Total Fat (gm)	% Calories from Fat	Total Calories
Flank, medium fat, stewed	——	90	32.3	75	390

SOURCES: *Composition of Foods: Beef Products—Raw. Processed. Prepared. Agriculture Handbook* 8-13. U.S. Department of Agriculture, Human Nutrition Information Service (August 1986).

Composition of Foods: Pork Products—Raw. Processed. Prepared. Agriculture Handbook 8-10. U.S. Department of Agriculture, Human Nutrition Information Service (August 1983).

Home and Garden Bulletin. Nutritive Value of Foods. No. 72. U.S. Department of Agriculture, Human Nutrition Information Service (1986).

Table 12
Poultry: Fat and Cholesterol Comparison Chart

Product (3½ oz, cooked)	Sat. Fat. (gm)	Chol. (mg)	Total Fat (gm)	% Calories from Fat	Total Calories
Turkey, fryer-roasters, light meat without skin, roasted	0.4	86	1.9	8	140
Chicken, roasters, light meat without skin, roasted	1.1	75	4.1	24	153
Turkey, fryer-roasters, light meat with skin, roasted	1.3	95	4.6	25	164

Table 12 (*Continued*)

Product (3½ oz, cooked)	Sat. Fat. (gm)	Chol. (mg)	Total Fat (gm)	% Calories from Fat	Total Calories
Chicken, broilers or fryers, light meat without skin, roasted	1.3	85	4.5	24	173
Turkey, fryer-roasters, dark meat without skin, roasted	1.4	112	4.3	24	162
Chicken, stewing, light meat without skin, stewed	2.0	70	8.0	34	213
Turkey, roll, light and dark	2.0	55	7.0	42	149
Turkey, fryer-roasters, dark meat with skin, roasted	2.1	117	7.1	35	182
Chicken, roasters, dark meat without skin, roasted	2.4	75	8.8	44	178
Chicken, broilers or fryers, dark meat without skin, roasted	2.7	93	9.7	43	205
Chicken, broilers or fryers, light meat with skin, roasted	3.0	85	10.9	44	222

Table 12 (*Continued*)

Product (3½ oz, cooked)	Sat. Fat. (gm)	Chol. (mg)	Total Fat (gm)	% Calories from Fat	Total Calories
Chicken, stewing, dark meat without skin, stewed	4.1	95	15.3	53	258
Duck, domesticated, flesh only, roasted	4.2	89	11.2	50	201
Chicken, broilers or fryers, dark meat with skin, roasted	4.4	91	15.8	56	253
Goose, domesticated, flesh only, roasted	4.6	96	12.7	48	238
Turkey, bologna, about 3½ slices	5.1	99	15.2	69	199
Chicken frankfurter, about 2	5.5	101	19.5	68	257
Turkey frankfurter, about 2	5.9	107	17.7	70	226

SOURCE: *Composition of Foods: Poultry Products—Raw. Processed. Prepared. Agriculture Handbook* 8-5. U.S. Department of Agriculture, Science and Education Administration (August 1979).

Fish and shellfish, in general, have a lot less saturated fat and cholesterol than meat and poultry. However, some shellfish is relatively high in cholesterol and should be eaten less often. Fish and shellfish also contain less total fat and calories than meat and poultry.

Table 13
Fish and Shellfish: Fat and Cholesterol Comparison Chart

Product (3½ oz, cooked)	Sat. Fat. (gm)	Chol. (mg)	Omega-III Fatty Acids (gm)	Total Fat (gm)	% Calories from Fat	Total Calories
Finfish						
Haddock, dry heat	0.2	74	0.2	0.9	7	112
Cod, Atlantic, dry heat	0.2	55	0.2	0.9	7	105
Pollock, walleye, dry heat	0.2	96	1.5	1.1	9	113
Perch, mixed species, dry heat	0.2	42	0.3	1.2	9	117
Grouper, mixed species, dry heat	0.3	47	——	1.3	10	118
Whiting, mixed species, dry heat	0.3	84	0.9	1.7	13	115
Snapper, mixed species, dry heat	0.4	47	——	1.7	12	128

Table 13 (*Continued*)

Product (3½ oz, cooked)	Sat. Fat. (gm)	Chol. (mg)	Omega-III Fatty Acids (gm)	Total Fat (gm)	% Calories from Fat	Total Calories
Halibut, Atlantic and Pacific, dry heat	0.4	41	0.6	2.9	19	140
Rockfish, Pacific, dry heat	0.5	44	0.5	2.0	15	121
Sea Bass, mixed species, dry heat	0.7	53	——	2.5	19	124
Trout, rainbow, dry heat	0.8	73	0.9	4.3	26	151
Swordfish, dry heat	1.4	50	1.1	5.1	30	155
Tuna, bluefin, dry heat	1.6	49	——	6.3	31	184
Salmon, sockeye, dry heat	1.9	87	1.3	11.0	46	216
Anchovy, European, canned	2.2	——	2.1	9.7	42	210
Herring, Atlantic, dry heat	2.6	77	2.1	11.5	51	203
Eel, dry heat	3.0	161	0.7	15.0	57	236
Mackerel, Atlantic, dry heat	4.2	75	1.3	17.8	61	262

Table 13 (*Continued*)

Product (3½ oz, cooked)	Sat. Fat. (gm)	Chol. (mg)	Omega-III Fatty Acids (gm)	Total Fat (gm)	% Calories from Fat	Total Calories
Pompano, Florida, dry heat	4.5	64	——	12.1	52	211
Crustaceans						
Lobster, northern	0.1	72	0.1	0.6	6	98
Crab, blue, moist heat	0.2	100	0.5	1.8	16	102
Shrimp mixed species, moist heat	0.3	195	0.3	1.1	10	99
Mollusks						
Whelk, moist heat	0.1	130	——	0.8	3	275
Clam, mixed species, moist heat	0.2	67	0.3	2.0	12	148
Mussel, blue, moist heat	0.9	56	0.8	4.5	23	172

Table 13 (*Continued*)

Product (3½ oz, cooked)	Sat. Fat. (gm)	Chol. (mg)	Omega-III Fatty Acids (gm)	Total Fat (gm)	% Calories from Fat	Total Calories
Oyster, Eastern, moist heat	1.3	109	1.0	5.0	33	137

SOURCE: *Composition of Foods: Finfish and Shellfish Products—Raw. Processed. Prepared. Agriculture Handbook* 8-15. U.S. Department of Agriculture (in press).

Whole milk dairy products are relatively high in saturated fat and cholesterol when compared ounce for ounce with meat, poultry, and seafood. In general, the hard cheeses are much higher in saturated fat and cholesterol than yogurt and most soft cheeses.

Table 14
Dairy and Egg Products: Fat and Cholesterol Comparison Chart

Product	Sat. Fat. (gm)	Chol. (mg)	Total Fat (gm)	% Calories from Fat	Total Calories
Milk (*8 oz*)					
Skim milk	0.3	4	0.4	5	86
Buttermilk	1.3	9	2.2	20	99
Low-fat milk (1% fat)	1.6	10	2.6	23	102
Low-fat milk (2% fat)	2.9	18	4.7	35	121
Whole milk (3.3% fat)	5.1	33	8.2	49	150

Table 14 (*Continued*)

Product	Sat. Fat. (gm)	Chol. (mg)	Total Fat (gm)	% Calories from Fat	Total Calories
Yogurt *(4 oz)*					
Plain, low-fat	0.1	2	0.2	3	63
Plain, regular	2.4	14	3.7	47	70
Cheese					
Cottage cheese, low-fat (1% fat), 4 oz	0.7	5	1.2	13	82
Mozzarella, part-skim, 1 oz	2.9	16	4.5	56	72
Cottage cheese, creamed, 4 oz	3.2	17	5.1	39	117
Mozzarella, 1 oz	3.7	22	6.1	69	80
Sour cream, 1 oz	3.7	12	5.9	87	61
American processed cheese spread, pasteurized, 1 oz	3.8	16	6.0	66	82
Feta, 1 oz	4.2	25	6.0	72	75
Neufchatel, 1 oz	4.2	22	6.6	81	74
Camembert, 1 oz	4.3	20	6.9	73	85
American processed cheese food, pasteurized, 1 oz	4.4	18	7.0	68	93
Provolone, 1 oz	4.8	20	7.6	68	100
Limburger, 1 oz	4.8	26	7.7	75	93
Brie, 1 oz	4.9	28	7.9	74	95
Romano, 1 oz	4.9	29	7.6	63	110
Gouda, 1 oz	5.0	32	7.8	69	101
Swiss, 1 oz	5.0	26	7.8	65	107
Edam, 1 oz	5.0	25	7.9	70	101
Brick, 1 oz	5.3	27	8.4	72	105

Table 14 (*Continued*)

Product	Sat. Fat. (gm)	Chol. (mg)	Total Fat (gm)	% Calories from Fat	Total Calories
Blue, 1 oz	5.3	21	8.2	73	100
Gruyere, 1 oz	5.4	31	9.2	71	117
Muenster, 1 oz	5.4	27	8.5	74	104
Parmesan, 1 oz	5.4	22	8.5	59	129
Monterey Jack, 1 oz	5.5	25	8.6	73	106
Roquefort, 1 oz	5.5	26	8.7	75	105
Ricotta, part-skim, 4 oz	5.6	25	9.0	52	156
American processed cheese, pasteurized, 1 oz	5.6	27	8.9	75	106
Colby, 1 oz	5.7	27	9.1	73	112
Cheddar, 1 oz	6.0	30	9.4	74	114
Cream cheese, 1 oz	6.2	31	9.9	90	99
Ricotta, whole milk, 4 oz	9.4	58	14.7	67	197
Eggs					
Egg, chicken, white	0	0	Trace	0	16
Egg, chicken, whole	1.7	274	5.6	64	79
Egg, chicken, yolk	1.7	272	5.6	80	63

SOURCE: *Composition of Foods: Dairy and Egg Products—Raw. Processed. Prepared. Agriculture Handbook* 8-1. U.S. Department of Agriculture, Agriculture Research Service (November 1976).

If you are trying to lose weight, the calories will be of special interest to you. Although some frozen desserts are lower in fat than others, they may be just as high in calories as the higher fat products because of their sugar content. You will usually want to select those desserts not only low in fat but also low in calories. Save those higher in calories for special treats.

Table 15

Frozen Desserts: Fat and Cholesterol Comparison Chart

Product (1 cup)	Sat. Fat. (gm)	Chol. (mg)	Total Fat (gm)	% Calories from Fat	Total Calories
Fruit popsicle, 1 bar	——	——	0.0	0	65
Fruit ice	——	——	Trace	0	247
Fudgsicle	——	——	0.2	2	91
Frozen yogurt, fruit-flavored	——	——	2.0	8	216
Sherbet, orange	2.4	14	3.8	13	270
Pudding pops, 1 pop	2.5	1	2.6	25	94
Ice milk, vanilla, soft serve	2.9	13	4.6	19	223
Ice milk, vanilla, hard	3.5	18	5.6	28	184
Ice cream, vanilla, regular	8.9	59	14.3	48	269
Ice cream, french vanilla, soft serve	13.5	153	22.5	54	377
Ice cream, vanilla, rich, 16% fat	14.7	88	23.7	61	349

SOURCES: *Composition of Foods: Dairy and Egg Products—Raw. Processed. Prepared. Agriculture Handbook* 8-1. U.S. Department of Agriculture, Agriculture Research Service (November 1976).

J. Pennington and H. Church, *Bowes and Church's Food Values of Portions Commonly Used* (14th ed. Philadelphia: J. B. Lippincott, 1985).

All fats and oils are high in calories, 115–120 calories per tablespoon.

Table 16

Fats and Oils: Comparison Chart

Product (1 Tbsp)	Sat. Fat. (gm)	Chol. (mg)	Polyunsaturated Fatty Acids (gm)	Mono-Unsaturated Fatty Acids (gm)
Rapeseed oil (canola oil)	0.9	0	4.5	7.6
Safflower oil	1.2	0	10.1	1.6
Sunflower oil	1.4	0	5.5	6.2
Peanut butter, smooth	1.5	0	2.3	3.7
Corn oil	1.7	0	8.0	3.3
Olive oil	1.8	0	1.1	9.9
Hydrogenated sunflower oil	1.8	0	4.9	6.3
Margarine, liquid, bottled	1.8	0	5.1	3.9
Margarine, soft, tub	1.8	0	3.9	4.8
Sesame oil	1.9	0	5.7	5.4
Soybean oil	2.0	0	7.9	3.2
Margarine stick	2.1	0	3.6	5.1
Peanut oil	2.3	0	4.3	6.2
Cottonseed oil	3.5	0	7.1	2.4
Lard	5.0	12	1.4	5.8
Beef tallow	6.4	14	0.5	5.3
Palm oil	6.7	0	1.3	5.0
Butter	7.1	31	0.4	3.3
Cocoa butter	8.1	0	0.4	4.5

Table 16 (*Continued*)

Product (1 Tbsp)	Sat. Fat. (gm)	Chol. (mg)	Polyunsaturated Fatty Acids (gm)	Mono-Unsaturated Fatty Acids (gm)
Palm kernel oil	11.1	0	0.2	1.5
Coconut oil	11.8	0	0.2	0.8

SOURCES: *Composition of Foods: Fats and Oils—Raw. Processed. Prepared. Agriculture Handbook* 8-4. U.S. Department of Agriculture, Science and Education Administration (June 1979).
Composition of Foods: Legumes and Legume Products—Raw. Processed. Prepared. Agriculture Handbook 8-16. U.S. Department of Agriculture, Human Nutrition Information Service (December 1986).

Most nuts and seeds would appear to be appropriate foods to eat because they contain little saturated fat. However, except for chestnuts, they are all high in total fat and consequently high in calories.

Table 17
Nuts and Seeds: Fat Comparison Chart

Product (1 oz)	Sat. Fat. (gm)	Chol. (mg)	Total Fat (gm)	% Calories from Fat	Total Calories
European chestnuts	0.2	0	1.1	9	105
Filberts or hazelnuts	1.3	0	17.8	89	179
Almonds	1.4	0	15.0	80	167
Pecans	1.5	0	18.4	89	187

Table 17 (*Continued*)

Product (1 oz)	Sat. Fat. (gm)	Chol. (mg)	Total Fat (gm)	% Calories from Fat	Total Calories
Sunflower seed kernels, roasted	1.5	0	1.4	77	165
English walnuts	1.6	0	17.6	87	182
Pistachio nuts	1.7	0	13.7	75	164
Peanuts	1.9	0	14.0	76	164
Hickory nuts	2.0	0	18.3	88	187
Pine nuts, pignolia	2.2	0	14.4	89	146
Pumpkin and squash seed kernels	2.3	0	12.0	73	148
Cashew nuts	2.6	0	13.2	73	163
Macadamia nuts	3.1	0	20.9	95	199
Brazil nuts	4.6	0	18.8	91	186
Coconut meat, unsweetened	16.3	0	18.3	88	187

SOURCES: *Composition of Foods: Legumes and Legume Products—Raw. Processed. Prepared. Agriculture Handbook* 8-16. U.S. Department of Agriculture, Human Nutrition Information Service (December 1986).

Composition of Foods: Nut and Seed Products—Raw. Processed. Prepared. Agriculture Handbook 8-12. U.S. Department of Agriculture, Human Nutrition Information Service (September 1984).

Table 18
Breads, Cereals, Pasta, Rice, and Dried Peas and Beans: Fat and Cholesterol Comparison Chart

Product	Sat. Fat. (gm)	Chol. (mg)	Total Fat (gm)	% Calories from Fat	Total Calories
Breads					
Melba toast, 1 plain	0.1	0	Trace	0	20
Pita, ½ large shell	0.1	0	1.0	5	165
Corn tortilla	0.1	0	1.0	14	65
Rye bread, 1 slice	0.2	0	1.0	14	65
English muffin	0.3	0	1.0	6	140
Bagel, 1, 3½" diameter	0.3	0	2.0	9	200
White bread, 1 slice	0.3	0	1.0	14	65
Rye krisp, 2 triple crackers	0.3	0	1.0	16	56
Whole wheat bread, 1 slice	0.4	0	1.0	13	70
Saltines, 4	0.5	4	1.0	18	50
Hamburger bun	0.5	Trace	2.0	16	115
Hot dog bun	0.5	Trace	2.0	16	115
Pancake, 1, 4" diameter	0.5	16	2.0	30	60
Bran muffin, 1, 2½" diameter	1.4	24	6.0	43	125
Corn muffin, 1, 2½" diameter	1.5	23	5.0	31	145
Plain doughnut, 1, 3¼" diameter	2.8	20	12.0	51	210
Croissant, 1, 4½" by 4"	3.5	13	12.0	46	235
Waffle, 1, 7" diameter	4.0	102	13.0	48	245

Table 18 (*Continued*)

Product	Sat. Fat. (gm)	Chol. (mg)	Total Fat (gm)	% Calories from Fat	Total Calories
Cereals (*1 cup*)					
Corn flakes	Trace	——	0.1	0	98
Cream of Wheat, cooked	Trace	——	0.5	3	134
Corn grits, cooked	Trace	——	0.5	3	146
Oatmeal, cooked	0.4	——	2.4	15	145
Granola	5.8	——	33.1	50	595
100% Natural Cereal with raisins and dates	13.7	——	20.3	37	496
Pasta (*1 cup*)					
Spaghetti, cooked	0.1	0	1.0	6	155
Elbow macaroni, cooked	0.1	0	1.0	6	155
Egg noodles, cooked	0.5	50	2.0	11	160
Chow mein noodles, canned	2.1	5	11.0	45	220
Rice (*1 cup cooked*)					
Rice, white	0.1	0	0.5	2	225
Rice, brown	0.3	0	1.0	4	230
Dried Peas and Beans (*1 cup cooked*)					
Split peas	0.1	0	0.8	3	231
Kidney beans	0.1	0	1.0	4	225
Lima beans	0.2	0	0.7	3	217

Table 18 (*Continued*)

Product	Sat. Fat. (gm)	Chol. (mg)	Total Fat (gm)	% Calories from Fat	Total Calories
Black eyes peas	0.3	0	1.2	5	200
Garbanzo beans	0.4	0	4.3	14	269

SOURCES: *Composition of Foods: Breakfast Cereals—Raw. Processed. Prepared. Agriculture Handbook* 8-8. U.S. Department of Agriculture, Human Nutrition Information Service (July 1982).

Composition of Foods: Legumes and Legume Products—Raw. Processed. Prepared. Agriculture Handbook 8-16. U.S. Department of Agriculture, Nutrition Monitoring Division (December 1986).

Home and Garden Bulletin. Nutritive Value of Foods. No. 72. U.S. Department of Agriculture, Human Nutrition Information Service (1986).

Since the foods in the following table may be sweet even if they are low in fat, they could be high in calories. Fruits, vegetables, and breads provide tasty low-fat, low-calorie alternatives.

Table 19
Sweets and Snacks: Fat and Cholesterol Comparison Chart

Product	Sat. Fat. (gm)	Chol. (mg)	Total Fat (gm)	% Calories from Fat	Total Calories
Beverages					
Ginger ale, 12 oz	0.0	0	0.0	0	125
Cola, regular, 12 oz	0.0	0	0.0	0	160
Chocolate shake, 10 oz	6.5	37	10.5	26	360
Candy (*1 oz*)					
Hard candy	0.0	0	0.0	0	110
Gum drops	Trace	0	Trace	Trace	100
Fudge	2.1	1	3.0	24	145
Milk chocolate	5.4	6	9.0	56	145

Table 19 (*Continued*)

Product	Sat. Fat. (*gm*)	Chol. (*mg*)	Total Fat (*gm*)	% Calories from Fat	Total Calories
Cookies					
Vanilla wafers 5 cookies, 1¾″ diameter	0.9	12	3.3	32	94
Fig bars, 4 cookies, 1⅝″ by 1⅝ by ⅔″	1.0	27	4.0	17	210
Chocolate brownie with icing, 1½″ by 1¾″ by ⅞″	1.6	14	4.0	36	100
Oatmeal cookies, 4 cookies, 2⅝″ diameter	2.5	2	10.0	37	245
Chocolate chip cookies, 4 cookies, 2¼″ diameter	3.9	18	11.0	54	185
Cakes and Pies					
Angel-food cake, 1/12 of 10″ cake	Trace	0	Trace	Trace	125
Gingerbread, 1/9 of 8″ cake	1.1	1	4.0	21	175
White layer cake with white icing, 1/16 of 9″ cake	2.1	3	9.0	32	260
Yellow layer cake with chocolate icing, 1/16 of 9″ cake	3.0	36	8.0	31	235

Table 19 (*Continued*)

Product	Sat. Fat. (gm)	Chol. (mg)	Total Fat (gm)	% Calories from Fat	Total Calories
Pound cake, ¹⁄₁₇ of loaf	3.0	64	5.0	41	110
Devil's food cake with chocolate icing, ¹⁄₁₆ of 9″ cake	3.5	37	8.0	31	235
Lemon meringue pie, ¹⁄₆ of 9″ pie	4.3	143	14.0	36	355
Apple pie, ¹⁄₆ of 9″ pie	4.6	0	18.0	40	405
Cream pie, ¹⁄₆ of 9″ pie	15.0	8	23.0	46	455
Snacks					
Popcorn, air-popped, 1 cup	Trace	0	Trace	Trace	30
Pretzels, stick, 2¼″, 10 pretzels	Trace	0	Trace	Trace	10
Popcorn with oil, salted, 1 cup	0.5	0	3.0	49	55
Corn chips, 1 oz.	1.4	25	9.0	52	155
Potato chips, 1 oz.	2.6	0	10.1	62	147
Pudding					
Gelatin	0.0	0	0.0	0	70
Tapioca, ½ cup	2.3	15	4.0	25	145
Chocolate pudding, ½ cup	2.4	15	4.0	24	150

SOURCE: *Home and Garden Bulletin. Nutritive Value of Foods.* No. 72. U.S. Department of Agriculture, Human Nutrition Information Service (1986).

Table 20
Miscellaneous Items: Fat and Cholesterol Comparison Chart

Product	Sat. Fat. (gm)	Chol. (mg)	Total Fat (gm)	% Calories from Fat	Total Calories
Gravies *(½ cup)*					
Au jus, canned	0.1	1	0.3	3	80
Turkey, canned	0.7	3	2.5	37	61
Beef, canned	1.4	4	2.8	41	62
Chicken, canned	1.7	3	6.8	65	95
Sauces *(½ cup)*					
Sweet and sour	Trace	0	0.1	< 1	147
Barbecue	0.3	0	2.3	22	94
White	3.2	17	6.7	50	121
Cheese	4.7	26	8.6	50	154
Sour cream	8.5	45	15.1	53	255
Hollandaise	20.9	94	34.1	87	353
Bearnaise	20.9	99	34.1	88	351
Salad Dressings *(1 Tbsp)*					
Russian, low-calorie	0.1	1	0.7	27	23
French, low-calorie	0.1	1	0.9	37	22
Italian, low-calorie	0.2	1	1.5	85	16
Thousand Island, low-calorie	0.2	2	1.6	59	24
Imitation mayonnaise	0.5	4	2.9	75	35
Thousand Island, regular	0.9	——	5.6	86	59
Italian, regular	1.0	——	7.1	93	69
Russian, regular	1.1	——	7.8	92	76
French, regular	1.5	——	6.4	86	67
Blue cheese	1.5	——	8.0	93	77
Mayonnaise	1.6	8	11.0	100	99

Table 20 (*Continued*)

Product	Sat. Fat. (gm)	Chol. (mg)	Total Fat (gm)	% Calories from Fat	Total Calories
Other					
Olives, green, 4 medium	0.2	0	1.5	90	15
Nondairy creamer, powdered, 1 teaspoon	0.7	0	1.0	90	10
Avocado, Florida	5.3	0	27.0	72	340
Pizza, cheese, ⅛ of 15″ diameter	4.1	56	9.0	28	290
Quiche Lorraine, ⅛ of 8″ diameter	23.2	285	48.0	72	600

SOURCES: *Composition of Foods: Fats and Oils—Raw. Processed. Prepared. Agriculture Handbook* 8-4. U.S. Department of Agriculture, Science and Education Administration (June 1979).
Composition of Foods: Soups, Sauces and Gravies—Raw. Processed. Prepared. Agriculture Handbook 8-6. U.S. Department of Agriculture, Science and Education Administration (February 1980).
Home and Garden Bulletin. Nutritive Value of Foods. No. 72. U.S. Department of Agriculture, Human Nutrition Information Service (1986).

B   *From Our Research Files*

Finally, before we leave you, here are some of our notes on that representative sampling of the research that taught us coronary heart disease can be prevented or reversed. Our emphasis here is on the mass of studies dealing with cholesterol; but as you will see, the other major modifiable risk factors are also discussed.

The battle against heart disease started with the lower animals, as do so many medical wars—chickens, rabbits, pigs, monkeys, cats, and dogs serving as stand-ins for their human counterparts. Such animal experiments *are* a naturally distressing concept for many people, yet the work has been vitally necessary, for the research has resulted in new medicines and procedures that have saved untold millions of human lives.

One of the earliest observations in the field of atherosclerosis research was made around the time of the Russian Revolution by a doctor named Anitschkow. He fed meat to rabbits and found that fat began accumulating in the walls of the animals' arteries. This led him to wonder what would happen if the rabbits were put back on their usual largely vegetarian diet. Two years later, having normalized their feeding, he found that the fatty deposits had dwindled. The notion had been born that clogged arteries could be cleared without some form of mechanical manipulation.

This discovery, like many other pioneering efforts, went largely unrecognized. It took two Americans, a generation later, to rediscover that atherosclerotic blockages could be produced in animals—this time chickens—by feeding them a diet rich in cholesterol. The obstructions in the arteries of some of the chickens melted away only ten weeks after the cholesterol feedings ended. This was monumentally important, for it meant that the long-held belief that atherosclerosis was irreversible was finally under attack.

The rabbit and chicken experiments weren't just a fluke. Later, more sophisticated experiments honed in on the vital concept of a critical cholesterol level, a kind of threshold below which the reversal process could be activated. The implications of this finding were enormous. Step by step, scientists came to the conclusion that when cholesterol levels fall to somewhere between 130 and 160, arteries begin to unclog. Soft, immature deposits seemed to dissolve more readily than older calcified ones; but clearly, reversal or regression was not only possible but documentable under the naked light of the microscope lamp.

More recently there have been new experiments with rabbits, concerning the now popular controversy over "good" HDL cholesterol and whether or not raising the level of HDL can actually have an impact on reversal of heart disease. In these current experiments, the rabbits were injected once a week with HDL cholesterol. They'd been on a high-cholesterol diet for twelve weeks. These injected rabbits actually showed regression, or reversal of the plaque formation in their arteries. This suggested that by artificially raising the high-density lipoprotein (HDL) level through the injection of HDL particles, fat can be removed from the arterial wall of the plaques, not only causing reversal but also preventing the plaque from rupturing.

There have also been recent experiments on pigs, in which

they've been placed on aspirin and Persantine (Persantine is a drug which, like aspirin, helps thin the blood). The outcome of these experiments? There was no progression of atherosclerosis for the treated pigs, as compared to those not treated with these medications.

Many studies have been conducted on various types of monkeys. In one, focused on Macaques and Rhesus monkeys for their cholesterol patterns, which are similar to those in human beings, M. L. Armstrong found that monkeys with blocked arteries, placed on a low-cholesterol diet, had reduced blockages. When the cholesterol was lowered to an average of 130–160 mg/dl, reversal of fatty and fibrous plaques occurred.

In another cholesterol study on monkeys over a twelve-month period, one group ate a 2% cholesterol diet and 25% coconut oil; a second group ate a 2% cholesterol diet and 25% Omega-III fish oil (for its blood-thinning effect), and coconut oil (ratio 1:1); and a third group ate a 2% cholesterol diet and 25% fish oil and coconut oil (ratio 3:1). Average serum cholesterol, group 1: 875; group 2: 463; group 3: 405. These findings showed that coconut oil and cholesterol increase degenerative changes in arterial walls. When the aorta and the carotid arteries were examined, the groups treated with Omega-III fatty acids showed much smaller amounts of plaque lesions, and fewer inflammatory cells in the plaque lesions, indicating an anti-inflammatory property of fish oil in preventing plaque formation.

Reading about animal experiments will probably never appeal to the vast majority of people, so although we could easily give you excerpts from many more, let us turn instead to the work done with humans. You know, from accompanying us through this book, that as the twentieth century progresses, so does the epidemic of coronary disease. The heart attack has presented itself as one of the unanticipated by-products of Western prosperity. It hasn't really taken very long to put two and two together: Lipids, which include fat and cholesterol, are linked to the process of atherosclerosis. And if reversal of clogged arteries could be achieved in lower animals, why couldn't the same be true in humans?

Pathologists, through coincidental observations, have often served as invaluable catalysts for medical progress. For example, it was during the dark days of World War I that a great German pathologist, Aschoff, began to notice changes in the appearance of the arteries of autopsied victims. With each passing year of trench warfare, as food supplies progressively dwindled, the fatty deposits appearing in the walls of major arteries became less and less common. Aschoff speculated that wartime deprivation and reversal of atherosclerosis might be tied together. At the time, though, he didn't see how this was possible.

Soviet pathologists after the siege of Leningrad in World War II, like Aschoff before them, found fewer and fewer atherosclerotic deposits in the victims' bodies.

In neighboring Finland, where the prewar death rate from heart attacks had been among the highest in the world, wartime food rationing also seemed to lead to a general decline in vascular disease.

What was this magic link between food and atherosclerosis? The most likely common denominator seemed to be cholesterol, whose levels understandably fell dramatically during periods of starvation.

The next step was to look, in a systematic way, at the association between cholesterol and atherosclerosis. This was undertaken in a massive fourteen-country effort, with a persistent pathologist named McGill coordinating the effort. Over 22,000 autopsies were performed, and the evidence showed conclusively that the higher the cholesterol level, the larger the area of atherosclerotic damage to the arteries.

By the 1970s, no serious student of the subject actively challenged the role of cholesterol and saturated fat in the development of atherosclerosis. But on the other hand, no one had yet managed to prove that, in humans, lowering blood levels of these lipids would in any way affect the course of coronary heart disease. Skeptics doubted the possibility of reversing deposits which, in most patients, had been building up in the arteries over decades.

Nevertheless, clinical trials were launched all over the world. The purpose of these studies was to answer just one question: Would bringing down cholesterol levels also bring down the numbers on coronary heart disease?

We now know that the answer is yes. Not only are prevention and stabilization of heart disease possible, but the combined weight of experimental and emerging human studies underscores the idea that blocked arteries can actually be unclogged, and this without any sort of mechanical intervention such as balloon or laser angioplasty. Coronary disease can be prevented or reversed by aggressively manipulating lipid levels.

The excess amount of cholesterol carried by LDL (low-density lipoprotein) is harmful, and crucial in the development of atherosclerotic lesions, but until recently it was not known how this cholesterol was deposited into the arteries. We now believe there is a biochemical event that transforms LDL cholesterol into an oxidized form likely to be taken up more easily by the scavenger cells in the artery wall. The LDL then contributes to plaque formation.

Oxidation is the chemical process by which substances are combined with oxygen. It is a normal process and occurs normally in body tissues. When we better understand the oxidation step of LDL cholesterol, it can potentially be manipulated by researchers so as to prevent atherosclerosis.

A recent study by Pekkaren and his colleagues showed that the risk of death by coronary artery disease for men with established coronary artery disease is tenfold greater than for men without elevated cholesterol or LDL levels. The risk is fourfold greater (still unacceptable) for men with no established coronary artery disease if they have elevated cholesterol levels versus normal cholesterol levels.

In reversing atherosclerosis, HDL cholesterol is more important than previously realized. This is the reason we treat it as an independent number that must be raised as LDL is lowered so that your total cholesterol factor balances out at zero.

But more vital than the actual level itself may be the turnover rate. Freshly synthesized HDL is a more active cholesterol scavenger than is HDL, which has already picked up cholesterol for transport to the liver. The point here is that if the production of new HDL can be increased, this would probably be more advantageous than simply increasing the total HDL level by other means.

The actual synthesis or production of new HDL is increased with the drug gemfibrozil and estrogens. Although low-fat diets can decrease the level of HDL, turnover studies show that these diets do not slow down its production. In other words, fresh HDL is being produced normally and is doing its job well. It is the old HDL that is being cleared away more effectively.

In the Helsinki Study, undertaken by the University of Helsinki in Finland, a cholesterol-lowering drug, gemfibrozil, was used to treat dyslipidemic men. An increase in HDL cholesterol was brought about by the gemfibrozil, and was associated with a decrease in coronary heart disease independent of the effect noted with a decline in LDL cholesterol. This showed HDL to be an independent factor in the total cholesterol picture. It helps fight coronary heart disease even when LDL is not lowered.

As you will see, much of the research has been initially based on studies using drug therapy. It was, in fact, a massive investigation of nearly 4,000 healthy men that smashed the last vestiges of doubt and suspicion surrounding the lipid hypothesis. Under the auspices of the multicenter Lipid Research Clinics, a randomized study tested the efficacy of cholesterol lowering in reducing the risk of coronary heart disease in middle-aged men who had no symptoms of heart disease but who were hypercholesterolemic. Candidates for the study had cholesterol levels over 265. They were randomly assigned to either a cholesterol-lowering group (using the drug cholestyramine) or a no-treatment group. Although cholesterol levels in the treated group fell by a mere 8%, the number of fatal and nonfatal heart attacks dropped by 19%.

Critics were quick to point out that the overall death rate, when taken by itself, didn't vary much between the two groups. Still, the study did manage to show convincingly that coronary heart disease could be favorably influenced by lowering cholesterol levels. And because it focused on apparently healthy men, it had tremendous implications for primary prevention—that is, neutralizing atherosclerosis before it can produce symptoms.

Another primary prevention trial, the Helsinki Study, assigned participants who were free of known coronary disease to either a treatment drug or a dummy pill. As little as two years after the study began, treated men became less prone to coronary disease. By the end of the study, the number of heart problems in the cholesterol-lowering group was 27.3 per 1,000, as opposed to 41.1 in the untreated group.

What about secondary prevention? Would reducing cholesterol levels in people with already-established heart disease be beneficial?

The Coronary Drug Project tried to answer this question. The Project was carried out as a collaborative study supported by research grants and other funds from the U.S. National Heart, Lung and Blood Institute. Over 1,000 male survivors of heart attacks were studied. Half were put on Niacin, a cholesterol-lowering vitamin. The others were given a placebo, or dummy pill. Nine years later, the death rate in the Niacin group was 11% lower than in the placebo group.

What accounted for this difference? Was the disease process merely brought to a halt, or did the atherosclerotic deposits actually begin to break down?

One way to find out was to use coronary angiograms. These show the coronary tree as it's filled with dye during heart catheterization. If the artery contains an obstruction, the channel of dye shows itself to be narrowed or blocked.

The U.S. National Heart, Lung and Blood Institute chose to use this technique to determine whether coronary artery narrowings were influenced by cholesterol-reducing treatment with the drug cholestyramine. After five years, when participants were recatheterized, blockages of 50% or more at the time of the first catheterization had progressed less in the patients on cholestyramine than in those without it.

Across the Atlantic, in the Netherlands, Dutch scientists used a computer to analyze the angiograms of patients who'd been on a vegetarian diet to bring down lipid levels. After only two years, no progression of the disease could be found in the arteries of those participants who'd managed the greatest change in their cholesterol makeup.

And what about reversal? Evidence that an anti-cholesterol program could actually unclog arteries emerged from CLAS, the Cholesterol-Lowering Atherosclerosis Study. Using Niacin and colestipol, LDL cholesterol was reduced by 26%, and HDL cholesterol increased by 37%. Angiograms showed that actual reversal could be seen in 16% of the treated patients after two years. After four years, reversal continued in 17% of the Niacin/colestipol group.

What type of coronary artery plaques can be expected to respond best to regression? It appears that plaques in the early stages of development with significant fat and cholesterol accumulation are the ones most likely to respond to reversal if proper methods are undertaken. This is particularly important since these plaques, though small, are the ones most likely to rupture and cause an acute heart attack. Affecting regression in such small, soft plaques is therefore extremely protective in preventing future heart attacks.

In a recently completed study, FATS, the impact of different cholesterol-lowering strategies versus dietary treatment was investigated. Reversal was most common in two aggressive drug regimens—those using Niacin and lovastatin (Mevacor).

Another two-and-a-half-year study on 136 subjects, all with coronary heart disease and hypercholesterolemia, found that by using a combination of a bile-acid sequestrant and lovastatin, a one-third incidence of regression was achieved. As you learned from the checkpoints, there will be times when such combination therapy is required.

We recently conducted a study with a colleague—Dr. Mark Matarazzo—in which 163 of our patients with high cholesterol values were treated with Niacin and lovastatin (Mevacor). Our study showed that Mevacor was much more effective in lowering LDL cholesterol than Niacin, and had much less liver toxicity. In fact, four of fifty-three patients treated with long-term Niacin therapy had an increase of three times normal their liver functions, requiring discontinuation of the Niacin. This was compared to only one out of 113 patients on Mevacor.

Both Niacin and Mevacor may be used long term for patients (our study followed them for over a year) as long as liver function tests are monitored. Mevacor seems to have less effect on the liver than Niacin, and both appear to be relatively safe if the patient is monitored carefully.

The evidence is clear and continues to mount. Bad lipids, like saturated fats and LDL cholesterol, contribute to the development of coronary disease. Lowering them can reduce the formation of atherosclerotic blockages that lead to coronary disease.

Let us take a moment here to tell you about lipoprotein(a). This substance has been found to be a marker predicting heart disease. Elevated levels have been associated with increased risk for heart disease or heart events such as stroke, heart attack, and coronary artery disease.

A high level of lipoprotein(a) in a young person is predictive of coronary disease, not only in that person but in the parents as well. Even when the total cholesterol is within the safe range, high lipoprotein(a) increases the risk of heart disease twofold.

Lipoprotein(a) bears a striking chemical resemblance to the clot-dissolving protein plasminogen. It is possible that lipoprotein(a) may even deposit cholesterol into a plaque that would otherwise be dissolved by plasminogen. This may be the genetic link we've been looking for.

In the context of genetics, let's spend some time discussing children and cholesterol. No race-related/age-related trends in lipid levels are apparent until age twelve, at which time a difference appears between black and white males in the form of a progressive increase for the white males in the ratio of LDL to HDL. That this phenomenon is exaggerated in young white males has important implications for earlier and greater development of coronary heart disease in white men. Young blacks show a stronger likelihood of developing hypertension.

By defining risk factor variables, we can identify children at high risk for cardiovascular problems, which makes it possible to tailor programs for such children, especially those with positive family histories. Children whose fathers have had heart attacks have abnormalities in their concentrations of Apo A-1 (apolipoprotein A-1 is the major protein of HDL) and Apo B (apolipoprotein B is the major protein of LDL and VLDL). Both can serve as important predictors of atherosclerotic cardiovascular disease. Those with such abnormalities are more likely to be white, older, cigarette smokers, and obese than children with healthy fathers.

The Bogalusa Heart Study (conducted in a biracial community, Bogalusa, Louisiana) was part of a program investigating the early development of atherosclerosis. We agree with the study's findings that every preschool child over two years of age should be screened, so that we are aware when lipoprotein intervention is necessary. This is our view despite the overall official recommendation to screen only those children at high

risk because of a known family history of dyslipidemia or premature coronary disease. Such a relatively limited screening
would fail to target from 20% to 50% of children with elevated
cholesterol.

The American Academy of Pediatrics guidelines for using
family history to identify children with high cholesterol were
studied in 117 children. Ninety-six of these children had a
fasting total cholesterol greater than 175 mg/dl; sixty-nine had
a fasting total cholesterol greater than 200 mg/dl.

So far as family histories were concerned, the families reported high cholesterol or premature heart attack, bypass surgery, or sudden cardiac death in a parent, grandparent, aunt, or
uncle (men less than fifty, women less than sixty).

Family history was negative in 21% of the children with
cholesterol greater than 175, and in 20% of those with total
cholesterol greater than 200.

As you can see, using family history alone as an indication
for cholesterol testing will result in failure to identify substantial numbers of children with high cholesterol levels. Children
should not be screened solely on the basis of their parent or
parents having a family history of high cholesterol, or if there is
a history of premature coronary disease in the family. Using
only these guidelines would miss 20% of those children with
elevated serum cholesterol levels.

Usually, diet and exercise can effectively treat hypercholesterolemia in children. After following a low-fat diet for three to
six months, if the cholesterol level is about 220 mg/dl and the
LDL level is above 160 mg/dl, and especially if there is a family
history of early heart disease, then drug therapy should be
started. The bile-acid sequestrants are the safest drugs. The
child should be at least of school age and healthy.

A study by Stein on children two to sixteen years of age
from high-risk families, using finger-stick cholesterol measure-
ments (which give only a *total* cholesterol number), identified
subjects with fasting cholesterol greater than 175. A total of

1,160 children were screened. Of these, 26% required a detailed lipid profile (lipoprotein analysis), and 7% were then referred for treatment. The majority responded to diet. However, 17% eventually were placed on a drug regimen.

It is vitally necessary for pediatrician, parents, and child to be informed of the potential for dietary or drug therapy as a treatment for dyslipidemia. Children should not consume more than 25–30% fat from their diet. Complex carbohydrates and vegetable proteins should make up the energy difference.

For those children with the highest levels of total cholesterol, dietary changes can produce an average reduction of 30 mg/dl. Using the Phase I diet of the American Heart Association (similar to the Philadelphia Formula Basic Heart Maintenance diet), Connor and Connor showed an 18-point drop in cholesterol. Using Phase II, there was a 39-point drop. Phase III (similar to the Philadelphia Formula Advanced Heart Repair diet) showed a drop of 53 mg/dl.

There is an ever-growing body of research not only on children and cholesterol but on women and coronary heart disease as well. Like men, some women are more at risk than others, and risk factors are cumulative. Let us share some of these findings with you.

When women undergo menopause, their HDL level begins declining, and total cholesterol and LDL eventually rise. These lipid abnormalities are favorably affected by hormone replacement therapy with estrogen. But there is significant controversy as to the exact nature of the hormone replacement. Recently, some studies have added small doses of progesterone to low-dose estrogen replacement therapy, to decrease the risk of endometrial and breast cancer. Further data is needed to assess the cardioprotective effect in these instances, and will surely be forthcoming.

If a woman has a history of smoking, high blood pressure, and high cholesterol, she raises her risk of heart disease eight times above that of a woman with none of these risk factors.

Those who have had early natural or surgically induced menopause (hysterectomy) have twice the risk of developing heart
disease as those at the same age who have not entered menopause. Older women are much more susceptible than younger
women to heart disease and are much more likely to develop
high blood pressure, high cholesterol, diabetes, and to be overweight as well.

The death rate for coronary heart disease is 19% higher, and
for stroke 79% higher, for black women than for white.

On average, heart disease manifests itself about ten years
later in women than in men. Actual heart attacks occur twenty
years later in women. A man with only one additional coronary
heart disease risk factor other than his sex, and an LDL greater
than 130, is considered to be at high risk. A woman with the
same cholesterol value must have two other risk factors to be at
high risk of coronary heart disease.

The Coronary Artery Surgery Study (CASS) was under-
taken at the Harold Brunn Institute, Mount Zion Hospital and
Medical Center, San Francisco; the Research Laboratories of St.
Joseph Hospital in Burbank, California; and the Department of
Epidemiology, School of Public Health, University of North
Carolina, Chapel Hill. The study showed smoking cessation to
lessen the risk of death or heart attack in both young and older
women.

High blood pressure is the single most important risk factor
for stroke. Even a mild elevation doubles the risk. Of the nearly
60 million Americans with high blood pressure, half are
women. High blood pressure is more common in black women
than in white. Oral contraceptives can raise blood pressure
levels.

Oral contraceptives also increase the risk of heart attack by
increasing body weight, altering blood clotting, and lowering
protective HDL. We will not recommend oral contraceptives if
a woman has a heart condition, has suffered a stroke, or has any
type of cardiovascular disease. Blood sugar changes dramati-

cally in women on these contraceptives, so that blood tests should be done periodically, especially if there's a family history of diabetes.

Both heart attack and stroke are more prevalent when women are overweight, and the overweight are more apt to have high blood cholesterol and high blood pressure as well.

Also, 85% of diabetics are at least 20% overweight. Both weight loss and increased physical activity are imperative. Diabetes is an independent risk factor for coronary heart disease, predisposing its victims to silent heart attacks. It is often called the women's disease, because after age forty-five about twice as many women as men develop adult-onset diabetes (which generally does not require insulin). Recently, in an article in the *New England Journal of Medicine,* it was reported that exercising effectively may protect against the emergence of this form of diabetes.

For reasons unknown, the risk of heart disease and heart-related deaths is much higher for diabetic women than for diabetic men. The occurrence of heart disease is doubled in these men, but tripled and quadrupled in women, especially prior to age fifty.

About fiber: For all of us—men, women, and children—research continues to prove that fiber (roughage) is necessary in a healthy diet. Until relatively recently, foods high in fiber had been pretty much purified out of our Western diet. This was unfortunate. Medical researchers have been finding that high-fiber diets prevent a whole spectrum of ills.

For example, researchers working in Africa have noted that Africans who consume a high-fiber diet have a lower incidence of coronary heart disease, hypertension, diabetes, and certain gastrointestinal disorders such as constipation, diverticulitis, hemorrhoids, appendicitis, cancer of the large bowel, and hiatal hernia.

Closer to home, Dr. Davidson and his colleagues out of Rush Medical Center studied adults for the cholesterol-lowering effects of oatmeal and oat bran. In this study, 156 adults with elevated cholesterol levels received either oatmeal or oat bran at doses of 28, 56, and 84 grams, or a control of 28 grams of farina, or oat bran or oatmeal containing the water-soluble fiber B glucan. (Farina is a fiber which lacks the B glucan.)

Patients followed a National Cholesterol Education Program Step I diet, which is a low-cholesterol diet, on the oatmeal, oat bran, and farina regimens.

After six weeks, there was a greater lowering of serum cholesterol levels for those taking the higher doses of oatmeal and oat bran than for those using farina. The farina did not significantly lower serum cholesterol. Oat bran was more effective in the test quantities than oatmeal. In fact, at high concentrations (56 to 84 grams, and 4 to 6 grams of B glucan respectively), oat bran lowered serum cholesterol by as much as 16%.

This data contrasts sharply with studies reported by several other researchers who have found no difference between the cholesterol-lowering effects of wheat bran and oat bran.

In a study published in 1988, University of California medical students were randomly given either oat bran or wheat bran. The students on daily doses of oat bran showed reductions in both their total cholesterol and bad LDL cholesterol levels, whereas those eating wheat bran didn't experience any change in their cholesterol levels at all. Also, a study published in 1990 showed oat bran to be more potent than oatmeal in lowering cholesterol in patients with hypercholesterolemia.

As you can see, the oat bran controversy must be considered unresolved.

Another controversy concerns alcohol. Numerous epidemiological studies support the fact that, to a certain point, there is an inverse relationship between alcohol consumption and the risk of coronary disease. One study published in *The Lancet* (August 1991) described how nearly 44,000 men were followed over a ten-year period. There were 21,000 men who drank less than 5 grams of alcohol a day, and 23,000 who drank between 5 and 30 grams of alcohol a day. The study noted that there were forty fewer cases of coronary disease over the ten-year period in those who drank moderately.

This was significant as a statistical difference; but for the real-life use of alcohol, as a method of preventing heart disease, the small benefits do not justify the risks. Alcohol has too many harmful effects. It can raise triglycerides, raise blood pressure, cause weakening of the heart muscle, and create innumerable social problems which, at the very least, will result in increased stress—a major risk factor for coronary heart disease.

Our focus in this postscript has been primarily on one major risk factor (cholesterol/diet) known to influence heart disease. If the modification of this alone can contribute to reversal, how much can be achieved by a comparable attack on all fronts?

In a recent study conducted by Dr. Dean Ornish, forty-eight patients with coronary disease were randomly assigned to either a control group or an experimental group, which then underwent alterations in lifestyle, consisting of a vegetarian-type diet, stopping smoking, stress management training, and moderate exercise.

After one year, twenty-nine patients required cardiac catheterization; but of those who had initial and follow-up catheterization in the experimental group, the average diameter of narrowing had regressed from 41.4 to 37.8%, whereas in the control group there was a progression of narrowing from 44.1 to 46.2%.

Coronary blood flow increased in the experimental group as it decreased in the control group. The experimental group's total adherence to lifestyle changes correlates strongly with changes in the narrowing of the coronary arteries and in the coronary flow rate.

Some notes on exercise: Many studies have documented the value of exercise for every aspect of living. That exercise actually can protect against coronary heart disease is no longer questioned. Surveys of such diverse people as London double-decker bus conductors, San Francisco longshoremen, active Harvard alumni, and mail carriers show that the higher the level of physical activity, the lower the cardiac death rate.

Exercise increases the good HDL cholesterol. In a study on joggers, those running an average of eleven miles per week had an HDL cholesterol level of 58 mg/dl, while the average for inactive men was only 43 mg/dl. Even with a less intense training program, you can anticipate a 10% increase in your HDL, and this improvement seems to occur even without weight loss or a change in diet.

Regular exercise retards atherosclerosis by enlarging the size of the arterial channels. Vigorous treadmill exercises with monkeys showed a reduction of the thickening of the arterial lining.

And some notes on stress: Psychological distress is most definitely a coronary risk factor. In studying the effects of stress on the atherosclerotic process, an interesting study involving certified public accountants found that their cholesterol levels increased by up to 100 mg/dl around tax season, even when their diet remained unchanged.

Chronic stress also causes elevations in cortisone, an anti-inflammatory substance produced by the adrenal glands. Such increases have been linked to atherosclerosis and coronary heart disease. In fact, one researcher has theorized that excesses of adrenaline and cortisone result from repeated cycles of stress, probably involving periods of hopelessness alternating with active but ineffective coping. This pattern of alternating events might explain the layered structure of atherosclerotic plaque.

Cardiologists have long appreciated that many coronary-prone patients have distinctive emotional responses and ways of coping with their environment. A psychological profile has emerged that is increasingly being recognized as a significant factor in the development of coronary heart disease.

Early clinical impressions described cardiac patients as "worriers" or "joyless strivers," but it was not until the Menningers undertook a comprehensive psychoanalytic study of hospitalized cardiac patients that a more specific trait emerged: suppressed anger. This tendency was confirmed by later investigators.

Nearly twenty-five years after the work of the Menningers appeared in the *American Heart Journal,* Friedman and Rosenman described a specific behavior pattern that could predict heart attacks in certain individuals. They called it Type A. The Type A personality has since become an icon of popular culture: the competitive, hard-driving man or woman on the fast track, under pressure to get things done yesterday, who eventually drops dead of a fatal heart attack.

There is actual scientific evidence to support this stereotype. The Western Collaborative Group Study found that Type A behavior carried twice the risk of coronary heart disease as its opposite, the Type B behavior pattern. Significantly, behavior modification techniques to temper the Type A pattern succeeded in reducing, by 50%, recurrent nonfatal heart attacks.

Of course the Type A hypothesis, like everything else, has its critics. In fact, a series of multicenter studies (MRFIT, AMIS, MPIP) did not identify a connection between Type A behavior and illness or death from coronary heart disease. This may have been due, in part, to a failure to arrive at an exact definition and identification of the Type A personality.

Also, the Honolulu Heart Study of 8,000 men did not show that a high-stress job increased the risk of coronary heart disease.

The effects of anxiety on atherosclerosis have been studied all over the world. For example, in England, 2,200 subjects utilized a questionnaire format. Those who were anxious or depressed turned out to have more abnormalities in their electrocardiograms than those whose outlook was more easygoing and positive.

In Sweden, it was found that women experiencing sustained emotional distress or sleep disturbances were more prone to angina or heart attacks.

In the United States, anxiety scores in men with two or more blocked coronary arteries were higher than those with less severe disease.

Researchers have devised several simple tests designed to provoke stress and raise anxiety levels so as to study the body's response to these situations. For example, one involved the tension-generating situation of being asked to do mental arithmetic involving serially subtracting 7 from a four-digit number; another utilized a simulated public speaking situation. In patients with coronary artery disease, such tasks produced evidence, by the use of a sophisticated technique called positron emission tomography, of reduced blood delivery to the heart muscle.

When patients were connected to portable continuous electrocardiogram recorders called Holter monitors, diary entries of tension or worry correlated with electrocardiographic changes suspicious for ischemia, or reduced blood flow.

When the motion of the heart was assessed using a sonar-like method called echocardiography, abnormalities appeared in coronary patients when they performed mental arithmetic.

Well, we really have to stop for now. The studies we've presented represent only the tip of the iceberg. We could easily go on forever for, as I'm sure you've guessed, we're fascinated by all of these inquiries into medical mysteries.

If you would like to read further on your own, please refer to the Suggested Readings and Selected References on pp. 267–80.

C Risk Factor Update Sheets

PHILADELPHIA FORMULA

Starting Numbers

$$\left[\frac{LDL}{10} - \frac{HDL}{5}\right] + 2\left[\frac{\text{\# OF PACKS}}{\text{PER DAY}}\right] + \text{EXERCISE SCORE} + \text{STRESS SCORE} + \frac{SBP - 130}{20} = \underline{\quad}$$

As you obtain your starting numbers from your cholesterol blood test, blood pressure test, smoking habits, level of exercise (use p. 235 to calculate how much exercise you get), and stress, jot them down next to the relevant headings, then enter them into the equation.

CHOLESTEROL: LDL _____ HDL _____
SMOKING [PACKS PER DAY]: _____
EXERCISE SCORE: _____
STRESS SCORE: _____
BLOOD PRESSURE: _____

$$\left[\frac{\quad}{10} - \frac{\quad}{5}\right] + 2\left[\frac{\quad}{\text{PER DAY}}\right] + \underline{\quad} + \underline{\quad} + \frac{\quad - 130}{20} = \underline{\quad}$$

CHOLESTEROL SCORE

(Your doctor will tell you these numbers when the results of your lipoprotein analysis are back.)

LDL _____   HDL _____

Starting Numbers

PERSONAL EXERCISE SCORE

Be honest about how much exercise you get. Are you a dedicated athlete, taking joy from the feel of strong muscles and sweat, and finding every opportunity to get out and test yourself; a moderately active individual who enjoys the surge of well-being exercise provides; only mildly active, with a tendency toward laziness and a wealth of excuses for not exerting yourself most of the time; or a totally sedentary couch potato? Give yourself a score of:

0 (Athletic)
You are probably burning 1,500
calories or more per week.   EXCELLENT ____

1 (Moderately Active—exercise 3–4
times a week)
You should be burning 1,000–
1,499 calories per week.   GOOD ____

2 (Only Mildly Active—exercise
1–2 times a week, or physical
work)
You probably burn only 500–999
calories per week.   FAIR ____

3 (Sedentary)
Unfortunately, you are burning
less than 500 calories per week.   POOR ____

Starting Numbers

PERSONAL STRESS SCORE

If the item applies to you, put an X in the space.

1. Major family change: death, marriage, pregnancy, retirement, divorce, separation?
2. Have you or a family member had a major injury, illness, or chronic health problems, been in an accident or a significant near-miss situation in the past six months?
3. Has this required extensive medical evaluation or hospitalization?
4. Do you assume primary responsibility for an ill or handicapped spouse, parent, sibling, or child?
5. Do you, or an immediate family member, have a major drug or alcohol problem?
6. Do you have a gambling problem?
7. Are you experiencing sexual difficulties?
8. Are you hard-driving, competitive: don't take time to relax, take vacations, or have hobbies?
9. Are you worried about finances?
10. Have you had a major financial or personal success recently, such as job promotion, big salary increase, winning the lottery, etc?
11. Has your financial situation become much worse, perhaps due to problems with your boss, or problems with your company due to lay-offs?
12. Are you significantly in debt and unable to make payments on time?
13. Has your spouse begun or quit work outside the home?

Starting Numbers

PERSONAL STRESS SCORE *(Continued)*

14. Do you have hostile feelings toward people at work or at home?
15. Are you starting or ending some additional education?
16. Have you recently moved to a new home, remodeled your house, or moved to a new area?
17. Are you having frequent premenstrual tension?
18. Are you experiencing a change in sleeping or eating habits?

_____ TOTAL   /3 = _____ STRESS SCORE

BLOOD PRESSURE SCORE

(Your doctor or the nurse will give you these numbers when you have your blood pressure taken.)

$$\frac{\text{Systolic BP} - 130}{20} = \underline{\hspace{2cm}}$$

(If the top number is negative, your score is zero. For example, say your systolic blood pressure is 130, or lower. 130 minus 130 equals 0. This would mean your top number is negative, because for the purposes of our formula, 0 or anything lower is negative—not a cause for concern. You would then record 0 for your blood pressure score.)

PHILADELPHIA FORMULA

Numbers after Six Weeks on the Program

$$\left[\frac{LDL}{10} - \frac{HDL}{5}\right] + 2\left[\frac{\text{\# OF PACKS}}{\text{PER DAY}}\right] + \text{EXERCISE SCORE} + \text{STRESS SCORE} + \frac{SBP - 130}{20} = \underline{\hspace{1cm}}$$

Jot your new numbers down next to the relevant headings, then enter them into the equation. Are you moving closer to zero?

CHOLESTEROL: LDL _____ HDL _____
SMOKING [PACKS PER DAY]: _____
EXERCISE SCORE: _____
STRESS SCORE: _____
BLOOD PRESSURE: _____

$$\left[\frac{}{10} - \frac{}{5}\right] + 2\left[\frac{}{\text{PER DAY}}\right] + \underline{} + \underline{} + \frac{ - 130}{20} = \underline{\hspace{1cm}}$$

CHOLESTEROL SCORE

LDL _____   HDL _____

Six Week Numbers

PERSONAL EXERCISE SCORE

0 (Athletic)
You are probably burning 1,500
calories or more per week.   EXCELLENT ____

1 (Moderately Active—exercise 3–4
times a week)
You should be burning 1,000–
1,499 calories per week.   GOOD ____

2 (Only Mildly Active—exercise
1–2 times a week, or physical
work)
You probably burn only 500–999
calories per week.   FAIR ____

3 (Sedentary)
Unfortunately, you are burning
less than 500 calories per week.   POOR ____

What form of exercise or combination of exercises
have you chosen?

Six Week Numbers

PERSONAL STRESS SCORE

If the item applies to you, put an X in the space.

1. Major family change: death, marriage, pregnancy, retirement, divorce, separation?
2. Have you or a family member had a major injury, illness, or chronic health problems, been in an accident or a significant near-miss situation in the past six months?
3. Has this required extensive medical evaluation or hospitalization?
4. Do you assume primary responsibility for an ill or handicapped spouse, parent, sibling, or child?
5. Do you, or an immediate family member, have a major drug or alcohol problem?
6. Do you have a gambling problem?
7. Are you experiencing sexual difficulties?
8. Are you hard-driving, competitive: don't take time to relax, take vacations, or have hobbies?
9. Are you worried about finances?
10. Have you had a major financial or personal success recently, such as job promotion, big salary increase, winning the lottery, etc?
11. Has your financial situation become much worse, perhaps due to problems with your boss, or problems with your company due to lay-offs?
12. Are you significantly in debt and unable to make payments on time?
13. Has your spouse begun or quit work outside the home?

Six Week Numbers

PERSONAL STRESS SCORE *(Continued)*

14. Do you have hostile feelings toward people at work or at home?
15. Are you starting or ending some additional education?
16. Have you recently moved to a new home, remodeled your house, or moved to a new area?
17. Are you having frequent premenstrual tension?
18. Are you experiencing a change in sleeping or eating habits?

_____ TOTAL   /3 = _____ STRESS SCORE
Have you chosen a stress reduction technique?

BLOOD PRESSURE SCORE

$$\frac{\text{Systolic BP} - 130}{20} = \underline{\hspace{2cm}}$$

242   *Appendices*

PHILADELPHIA FORMULA

After Twelve Weeks (Three Months) on the Program

$$\left[\frac{LDL}{10} - \frac{HDL}{5}\right] + 2\left[\frac{\text{\# OF PACKS}}{\text{PER DAY}}\right] + \underset{\text{SCORE}}{\text{EXERCISE}} + \underset{\text{SCORE}}{\text{STRESS}} + \frac{SBP - 130}{20} = \underline{\quad}$$

Jot your new numbers down next to the relevant headings, then enter them into the equation. Are you moving closer to zero?

CHOLESTEROL: LDL _____ HDL _____
SMOKING [PACKS PER DAY]: _____
EXERCISE SCORE: _____
STRESS SCORE: _____
BLOOD PRESSURE: _____

$$\left[\frac{}{10} - \frac{}{5}\right] + 2\left[\frac{}{\text{PER DAY}}\right] + \underline{\quad} + \underline{\quad} + \frac{-130}{20} = \underline{\quad}$$

CHOLESTEROL SCORE

LDL _____   HDL _____

Three Month Numbers

PERSONAL EXERCISE SCORE

0 (Athletic)
You are probably burning 1,500
calories or more per week.   EXCELLENT ____

1 (Moderately Active—exercise 3–4
times a week)
You should be burning 1,000–
1,499 calories per week.   GOOD ____

2 (Only Mildly Active—exercise
1–2 times a week, or physical
work)
You probably burn only 500–999
calories per week.   FAIR ____

3 (Sedentary)
Unfortunately, you are burning
less than 500 calories per week.   POOR ____

How are you doing? Are you feeling better?

Three Month Numbers

PERSONAL STRESS SCORE

If the item applies to you, put an X in the space.

1. Major family change: death, marriage, pregnancy, retirement, divorce, separation?
2. Have you or a family member had a major injury, illness, or chronic health problems, been in an accident or a significant near-miss situation in the past six months?
3. Has this required extensive medical evaluation or hospitalization?
4. Do you assume primary responsibility for an ill or handicapped spouse, parent, sibling, or child?
5. Do you, or an immediate family member, have a major drug or alcohol problem?
6. Do you have a gambling problem?
7. Are you experiencing sexual difficulties?
8. Are you hard-driving, competitive: don't take time to relax, take vacations, or have hobbies?
9. Are you worried about finances?
10. Have you had a major financial or personal success recently, such as job promotion, big salary increase, winning the lottery, etc?
11. Has your financial situation become much worse, perhaps due to problems with your boss, or problems with your company due to lay-offs?
12. Are you significantly in debt and unable to make payments on time?
13. Has your spouse begun or quit work outside the home?

Three Month Numbers

PERSONAL STRESS SCORE *(Continued)*

14. Do you have hostile feelings toward people at work or at home?
15. Are you starting or ending some additional education?
16. Have you recently moved to a new home, remodeled your house, or moved to a new area?
17. Are you having frequent premenstrual tension?
18. Are you experiencing a change in sleeping or eating habits?

_____ TOTAL   /3 = _____ STRESS SCORE

Is your score at this checkpoint lower than your starting number?

BLOOD PRESSURE SCORE

$$\frac{\text{Systolic BP} - 130}{20} = \underline{\hspace{1cm}}$$

PHILADELPHIA FORMULA

After Eighteen Weeks on the Program

$$\left[\frac{LDL}{10} - \frac{HDL}{5}\right] + 2\left[\frac{\#\ OF\ PACKS}{PER\ DAY}\right] + \begin{array}{c}EXERCISE\\SCORE\end{array} + \begin{array}{c}STRESS\\SCORE\end{array} + \frac{SBP - 130}{20} = \underline{\quad}$$

Jot your new numbers down next to the relevant headings, then enter them into the equation. Are you moving closer to zero?

CHOLESTEROL: LDL _____ HDL _____
SMOKING [PACKS PER DAY]: _____
EXERCISE SCORE: _____
STRESS SCORE: _____
BLOOD PRESSURE: _____

$$\left[\frac{\quad}{10} - \frac{\quad}{5}\right] + 2\left[\frac{\quad}{PER\ DAY}\right] + \underline{\ } + \underline{\ } + \frac{\quad - 130}{20} = \underline{\quad}$$

CHOLESTEROL SCORE

LDL _____   HDL _____

Eighteen Week Numbers

PERSONAL EXERCISE SCORE

0 (Athletic)
You are probably burning 1,500
calories or more per week.   EXCELLENT ____

1 (Moderately Active—exercise 3–4
times a week)
You should be burning 1,000–
1,499 calories per week.   GOOD ____

2 (Only Mildly Active—exercise
1–2 times a week, or physical
work)
You probably burn only 500–999
calories per week.   FAIR ____

3 (Sedentary)
Unfortunately, you are burning
less than 500 calories per week.   POOR ____

If you're happy with your chosen form of exercise,
simply continue. If you're feeling bored with only one
type of exercise, remember, it's perfectly all right to combine different types. The only important thing is to keep
going, to keep trying to bring your exercise risk factor
score toward zero.

Eighteen Week Numbers

PERSONAL STRESS SCORE

If the item applies to you, put an X in the space.

1. Major family change: death, marriage, pregnancy, retirement, divorce, separation?
2. Have you or a family member had a major injury, illness, or chronic health problems, been in an accident or a significant near-miss situation in the past six months?
3. Has this required extensive medical evaluation or hospitalization?
4. Do you assume primary responsibility for an ill or handicapped spouse, parent, sibling, or child?
5. Do you, or an immediate family member, have a major drug or alcohol problem?
6. Do you have a gambling problem?
7. Are you experiencing sexual difficulties?
8. Are you hard-driving, competitive: don't take time to relax, take vacations, or have hobbies?
9. Are you worried about finances?
10. Have you had a major financial or personal success recently, such as job promotion, big salary increase, winning the lottery, etc?
11. Has your financial situation become much worse, perhaps due to problems with your boss, or problems with your company due to lay-offs?
12. Are you significantly in debt and unable to make payments on time?
13. Has your spouse begun or quit work outside the home?

Eighteen Week Numbers

PERSONAL STRESS SCORE *(Continued)*

14. Do you have hostile feelings toward people at work or at home?
15. Are you starting or ending some additional education?
16. Have you recently moved to a new home, remodeled your house, or moved to a new area?
17. Are you having frequent premenstrual tension?
18. Are you experiencing a change in sleeping or eating habits?

_____ TOTAL   /3 = _____ STRESS SCORE

Is your chosen method of relaxation bringing your stress risk factor score closer to zero?

BLOOD PRESSURE SCORE

$$\frac{\text{Systolic BP} - 130}{20} = \underline{\hspace{2cm}}$$

PHILADELPHIA FORMULA

After Twenty-four Weeks (Six Months) on the Program

$$\left[\frac{LDL}{10} - \frac{HDL}{5} \right] + 2\left[\frac{\text{\# OF PACKS}}{\text{PER DAY}} \right] + \frac{\text{EXERCISE}}{\text{SCORE}} + \frac{\text{STRESS}}{\text{SCORE}} + \frac{SBP - 130}{20} = \underline{\quad}$$

Jot your new numbers down next to the relevant headings, then enter them into the equation. Are you moving closer to zero?

CHOLESTEROL: LDL _____ HDL _____
SMOKING [PACKS PER DAY]: _____
EXERCISE SCORE: _____
STRESS SCORE: _____
BLOOD PRESSURE: _____

$$\left[\frac{}{10} - \frac{}{5} \right] + 2\left[\frac{}{\text{PER DAY}} \right] + \underline{\ } + \underline{\ } + \frac{- 130}{20} = \underline{\quad}$$

CHOLESTEROL SCORE

LDL _____   HDL _____

Six Month Numbers

PERSONAL EXERCISE SCORE

0 (Athletic)
You are probably burning 1,500
calories or more per week.   EXCELLENT ____

1 (Moderately Active—exercise 3–4
times a week)
You should be burning 1,000–
1,499 calories per week.   GOOD ____

2 (Only Mildly Active—exercise
1–2 times a week, or physical
work)
You probably burn only 500–999
calories per week.   FAIR ____

3 (Sedentary)
Unfortunately, you are burning
less than 500 calories per week.   POOR ____

    If you still have not improved your exercise score, and
especially if you started at, and remain at 3, you are simply not trying. It's vitally important for you to get enough
exercise. Don't imagine that it's enough just to improve in
one area, like diet, without trying to get to zero in each
category. As we told you from the beginning, this is a
comprehensive program, and it's for life.

Six Month Numbers

PERSONAL STRESS SCORE

If the item applies to you, put an X in the space.

1. Major family change: death, marriage, pregnancy, retirement, divorce, separation?
2. Have you or a family member had a major injury, illness, or chronic health problems, been in an accident or a significant near-miss situation in the past six months?
3. Has this required extensive medical evaluation or hospitalization?
4. Do you assume primary responsibility for an ill or handicapped spouse, parent, sibling, or child?
5. Do you, or an immediate family member, have a major drug or alcohol problem?
6. Do you have a gambling problem?
7. Are you experiencing sexual difficulties?
8. Are you hard-driving, competitive: don't take time to relax, take vacations, or have hobbies?
9. Are you worried about finances?
10. Have you had a major financial or personal success recently, such as job promotion, big salary increase, winning the lottery, etc?
11. Has your financial situation become much worse, perhaps due to problems with your boss, or problems with your company due to lay-offs?
12. Are you significantly in debt and unable to make payments on time?
13. Has your spouse begun or quit work outside the home?

Six Month Numbers

PERSONAL STRESS SCORE *(Continued)*

14. Do you have hostile feelings toward people at work or at home?
15. Are you starting or ending some additional education?
16. Have you recently moved to a new home, remodeled your house, or moved to a new area?
17. Are you having frequent premenstrual tension?
18. Are you experiencing a change in sleeping or eating habits?

_____ TOTAL   /3 = _____ STRESS SCORE

You're more than halfway through the nine-month countdown. How are you doing? How close are you getting down to zero?

BLOOD PRESSURE SCORE

$$\frac{\text{Systolic BP} - 130}{20} = \underline{\hspace{2cm}}$$

PHILADELPHIA FORMULA

After Thirty Weeks on the Program

$$\left[\frac{LDL}{10} - \frac{HDL}{5}\right] + 2\left[\frac{\text{\# OF PACKS}}{\text{PER DAY}}\right] + \text{EXERCISE SCORE} + \text{STRESS SCORE} + \frac{SBP - 130}{20} = \underline{\quad}$$

Jot your new numbers down next to the relevant headings, then enter them into the equation. Are you moving closer to zero?

CHOLESTEROL: LDL _____ HDL _____
SMOKING [PACKS PER DAY]: _____
EXERCISE SCORE: _____
STRESS SCORE: _____
BLOOD PRESSURE: _____

$$\left[\frac{}{10} - \frac{}{5}\right] + 2\left[\frac{}{\text{PER DAY}}\right] + \underline{\quad} + \underline{\quad} + \frac{\underline{\quad} - 130}{20} = \underline{\quad}$$

CHOLESTEROL SCORE

LDL _____   HDL _____

Thirty Week Numbers

PERSONAL EXERCISE SCORE

0 (Athletic)
You are probably burning 1,500
calories or more per week.   EXCELLENT ____

1 (Moderately Active—exercise 3–4
times a week)
You should be burning 1,000–
1,499 calories per week.   GOOD ____

2 (Only Mildly Active—exercise
1–2 times a week, or physical
work)
You probably burn only 500–999
calories per week.   FAIR ____

3 (Sedentary)
Unfortunately, you are burning
less than 500 calories per week.   POOR ____

Did the pep talk help at the last checkpoint? How
close are you getting to zero in your exercise score?

Thirty Week Numbers

PERSONAL STRESS SCORE

If the item applies to you, put an X in the space.

1. Major family change: death, marriage, pregnancy, retirement, divorce, separation?
2. Have you or a family member had a major injury, illness, or chronic health problems, been in an accident or a significant near-miss situation in the past six months?
3. Has this required extensive medical evaluation or hospitalization?
4. Do you assume primary responsibility for an ill or handicapped spouse, parent, sibling, or child?
5. Do you, or an immediate family member, have a major drug or alcohol problem?
6. Do you have a gambling problem?
7. Are you experiencing sexual difficulties?
8. Are you hard-driving, competitive: don't take time to relax, take vacations, or have hobbies?
9. Are you worried about finances?
10. Have you had a major financial or personal success recently, such as job promotion, big salary increase, winning the lottery, etc?
11. Has your financial situation become much worse, perhaps due to problems with your boss, or problems with your company due to lay-offs?
12. Are you significantly in debt and unable to make payments on time?
13. Has your spouse begun or quit work outside the home?

Thirty Week Numbers

PERSONAL STRESS SCORE *(Continued)*

14. Do you have hostile feelings toward people at work or at home?
15. Are you starting or ending some additional education?
16. Have you recently moved to a new home, remodeled your house, or moved to a new area?
17. Are you having frequent premenstrual tension?
18. Are you experiencing a change in sleeping or eating habits?

_____ TOTAL /3 = _____ STRESS SCORE

You're almost at the nine-month checkpoint. Only six more weeks to go. You should be closing in on zero now. How are you doing?

BLOOD PRESSURE SCORE

$$\frac{\text{Systolic BP} - 130}{20} = \underline{\hspace{1cm}}$$

PHILADELPHIA FORMULA

After Thirty-six Weeks (Nine Months) on the Program

$$\left[\frac{LDL}{10} - \frac{HDL}{5}\right] + 2\left[\frac{\text{\# OF PACKS}}{\text{PER DAY}}\right] + \text{EXERCISE SCORE} + \text{STRESS SCORE} + \frac{SBP - 130}{20} = \underline{\quad}$$

Jot your new numbers down next to the relevant headings, then enter them into the equation. Are you moving closer to zero?

CHOLESTEROL: LDL _____ HDL _____
SMOKING [PACKS PER DAY]: _____
EXERCISE SCORE: _____
STRESS SCORE: _____
BLOOD PRESSURE: _____

$$\left[\frac{\quad}{10} - \frac{\quad}{5}\right] + 2\left[\frac{\quad}{\text{PER DAY}}\right] + \underline{\quad} + \underline{\quad} + \frac{\quad - 130}{20} = \underline{\quad}$$

CHOLESTEROL SCORE

LDL _____   HDL _____

Nine Month Numbers

PERSONAL EXERCISE SCORE

0 (Athletic)
You are probably ɔurning 1,500
calories or more per week.   EXCELLENT ____

1 (Moderately Active—exercise 3–4
times a week)
You should be burning 1,000–
1,499 calories per week.   GOOD ____

2 (Only Mildly Active—exercise
1–2 times a week, or physical
work)
You probably burn only 500–999
calories per week.   FAIR ____

3 (Sedentary)
Unfortunately, you are burning
less than 500 calories per week.   POOR ____

Congratulations! Even if your exercise score has not zeroed out, you have at least stuck to the program. This nine-month checkpoint is not an ending. The Philadelphia Formula Nine-Month Countdown Program uses the nine-month final checkpoint because at this point you're on your own. After nine months of following the program, all of its separate facets should have fashioned some real changes in your lifestyle.

You've made it your new way of life.

Continue working to get your scores down to zero, if they are not already there. If they are zeroed out, double congratulations. But again, that's not an ending. Now you must keep them there.

Nine Month Numbers

PERSONAL STRESS SCORE

If the item applies to you, put an X in the space.

1. Major family change: death, marriage, pregnancy, retirement, divorce, separation?
2. Have you or a family member had a major injury, illness, or chronic health problems, been in an accident or a significant near-miss situation in the past six months?
3. Has this required extensive medical evaluation or hospitalization?
4. Do you assume primary responsibility for an ill or handicapped spouse, parent, sibling, or child?
5. Do you, or an immediate family member, have a major drug or alcohol problem?
6. Do you have a gambling problem?
7. Are you experiencing sexual difficulties?
8. Are you hard-driving, competitive: don't take time to relax, take vacations, or have hobbies?
9. Are you worried about finances?
10. Have you had a major financial or personal success recently, such as job promotion, big salary increase, winning the lottery, etc?
11. Has your financial situation become much worse, perhaps due to problems with your boss, or problems with your company due to lay-offs?
12. Are you significantly in debt and unable to make payments on time?
13. Has your spouse begun or quit work outside the home?

Nine Month Numbers

PERSONAL STRESS SCORE *(Continued)*

14. Do you have hostile feelings toward people at work or at home?
15. Are you starting or ending some additional education?
16. Have you recently moved to a new home, remodeled your house, or moved to a new area?
17. Are you having frequent premenstrual tension?
18. Are you experiencing a change in sleeping or eating habits?

_____ TOTAL   /3 = _____ STRESS SCORE

You've made it all the way through the nine-month program. What is your stress score? Have you made it to zero?

BLOOD PRESSURE SCORE

$$\frac{\text{Systolic BP} - 130}{20} = \underline{\hspace{2cm}}$$

Glossary

adrenaline (*n.*) a hormone (epinephrine) of the adrenal medulla that acts as a powerful stimulant in times of fear or arousal.

aerobic (*adj.*) living, active, or occurring only in the presence of oxygen.

angiogram (*n.*) an X-ray film of arteries obtained as they are injected with contrast dye.

angioplasty (*n.*) dilation of a vascular obstruction using an expandable balloon catheter.

arrhythmia (*n.*) abnormal heartbeat rhythm, caused by drugs, disease, the body's physiology, or a combination of factors.

atheroma (*n.*) fat deposit inside the lining of a blood vessel.

atherosclerosis (*n.*) an abnormal hardening within the arteries as the result of plaque formation.

bile acid (*n.*) substance secreted by the liver that aids in digestion.

bypass graft (*n.*) natural or synthetic tube used to bypass vascular obstructions.

cardiac catheterization (*n.*) an invasive test requiring the insertion of catheters into arteries and veins and subsequent dye injection to outline the coronary arteries for blockages.

catecholamine (*n.*) any of a group of chemicals produced in the adrenal gland and also synthetically for use as drugs, which function in the body's response to stress.

cholesterol (*n.*) a complex chemical present in all animal fats and widespread in the body, forming deposits in blood vessels.

coronary artery (*n.*) one of the arteries that supply the heart muscle with blood.

coronary thrombosis (*n.*) the formation of a blood clot (thrombus) in a coronary artery.

diastolic (*adj.*) diastolic blood pressure (DBP) is the lowest point to which the pressure drops between beats (contractions) of the heart, during which the chambers widen and fill with blood.

dyslipidemia (*n.*) an abnormal concentration of LDL, VLDL, or HDL cholesterol.

endothelium (*n.*) cells lining the inside of an artery wall.

exercise (*n.*) bodily exertion for the sake of developing and maintaining physical fitness.

fiber (*n.*) food content (cellulose) that adds roughage to the diet.

fibrinogen (*n.*) a protein present in blood plasma, essential to the process of blood coagulation.

fibrosis (*n.*) abnormal formation of fibrous tissue.

hemorrhoid (*n.*) swelling of a vein or veins in the lower rectum or anus.

high-density lipoprotein (HDL) cholesterol (*n.*) the "good" cholesterol, which is involved in reverse transport of fats out of the artificial wall of the liver.

hyperlipidemia   (*n.*) excessive quantity of fat in the blood.

hypertension   (*n.*) a common disorder, often with no symptoms, in which the blood pressure is persistently above 140/90 mg Hg. Obesity, hypercholesterolemia, and high sodium levels are some predisposing factors.

hypotension   (*n.*) blood pressure that is abnormally low, possibly resulting from hemorrhage, excessive fluid loss, heart malfunction, etc.

interferon   (*n.*) a naturally occurring anti-viral substance.

intima   (*n.*) the innermost part of a blood vessel wall.

ischemia   (*n.*) decreased blood supply to a given body part.

left ventricle   (*n.*) the left part of the heart, which does the major pumping.

lipids   (*n.*) blood fats.

lipoprotein   (*n.*) protein transport particle for cholesterol.

low-density lipoprotein (LDL) cholesterol   (*n.*) the "bad" cholesterol, which is deposited in the artery wall.

metabolic rate   (*n.*) the body's ability to burn calories.

mono-unsaturated fat   (*n.*) the "good" fats found in peanut oil, olive oil, and canola (rapeseed) oil, which do not raise serum cholesterol.

myocardial infarction   (*n.*) a heart attack; irreversible damage to the heart muscle usually caused by closure of a coronary artery or its branches.

nicotinic acid (niacin)   (*n.*) a vitamin of the B complex group, essential for normal function of the nervous system and gastrointestinal tract.

nutrition   (*n.*) the steps by which a living organism uses food for growth and replacement of tissue.

obesity (*n.*) a condition characterized by excessive bodily fat.

Omega-III fatty acids (*n.*) long chains of polyunsaturated fatty acids that enter the food chain when marine algae are eaten by cold-water fish.

plaque (*n.*) a cobblestonelike deposit (atheroma) inside the blood vessel's lining.

platelets (*n.*) particles in the blood which clump together and facilitate clotting.

polyunsaturated fat (*n*) the "good" fats found in corn, sunflower, safflower, soybean, and cottonseed oils, which do not raise serum cholesterol.

regression (*n.*) a return or reversal to a previous condition or state. (In treating heart disease, the best possible condition.)

saturated fat (*n.*) a fatty acid found chiefly in animal fats.

sequestrant (*n.*) a chemical that promotes the inhibition of normal ion behavior.

silent ischemia (*n.*) the phenomenon of no angina despite laboratory evidence of lack of heart circulation.

systolic (*adj.*) systolic blood pressure (SBP) refers to the pressure at the height of the pulse wave, caused by contraction of the heart, especially of the ventricles, driving blood into the aorta and pulmonary artery.

tachycardia (*n.*) an abnormally rapid heart rate—in an adult, over 100 beats per minute.

thrombus (*n.*) a blood clot attached to the interior wall of a vein or artery.

tissue plasminogen activator (TPA) (*n.*) a clot-dissolving substance produced by the body which may also be given as a drug to patients during a heart attack.

triglyceride (*n.*) a compound consisting of a fatty acid and glycerol that is the principal lipid in the blood.

ventricular fibrillation   (*n.*) a serious disturbance in cardiac rhythm, characterized by disorganized impulse conduction and ventricular contraction.

very low-density lipoprotein (VLDL) cholesterol   (*n.*) another form of lipoprotein, which takes on some of the bad cholesterol absorbed by HDL and transports it, and triglycerides, to the liver.

Suggested Readings and
Selected References

Abelin, T., Buehler, A., Muller, P., Vesanen, K., Imhof, P. R. "Controlled trial of transdermal nicotine patch in tobacco withdrawal." *The Lancet.* 1(8628):7–10, January 7, 1989.

Akerstedt, T., Gillberg, M., Hjemdahl, P., et al. "Comparison of urinary and plasma catecholamine responses to mental stress." *Acta Physiologica Scandinavica.* 117(1):19–26, January 1983.

Alfredsson, L., Karasek, R., Theorell, T. "Myocardial infarction risk and psychosocial work environment: An analysis of the male Swedish working force." *Social Science and Medicine.* 16(4):463–67, 1982.

Anitschkow, N. A History of Experimentation on Arterial Atherosclerosis in Animals. In E. V. Cowdry, ed., *Arteriosclerosis: A Survey of the Problem.* New York: Macmillan, 1967.

Armstrong, M. L., Megan, M. B. "Arterial fibrous proteins in cynomolgus monkeys after atherogenic and regression diets." *Circulation Research.* 36(2):256–61, February 1975.

Arntzenius, A. C., et al. "Diet, lipoproteins, and the progression of coronary atherosclerosis: The Leiden Intervention Trial." *New England Journal of Medicine.* 312(13):805–11, March 28, 1985.

Aschoff, L. *Lectures in Pathology* (Delivered in the United States, 1924). New York: Hoeber, 1924.

[Anonymous.] "Aspirin for heart patients." *FDA Drug Bulletin.* 15(4):34–36, December 1985.

Atterhog, J. H., Eliasson, K., Hjemdahl, P. "Sympathoadrenal and cardiovascular responses to mental stress, isometric handgrip, and cold pressor test in asymptomatic young men with primary T-wave abnormalities in the electrocardiogram." *British Heart Journal.* 46(3):311–19, September 1981.

Bagga, O. P., Gandhi, A. "A comparative study of the effect of Transcendental Meditation (T.M.) and Shavasana practice on the cardiovascular system." *Indian Heart Journal.* 35(1):39–45, January–February 1983.

Barboriak, J. J., Pintar, K., Van Horn, D., et al. "Pathologic findings in the aortocoronary vein grafts: A scanning electron microscope study." *Atherosclerosis.* 29(1):69–80, January 1978.

Benson, H. *The Relaxation Response.* New York: William Morrow, 1975.

Bevans, M., Davidson, J. D., Kendall, F. E. "Regression of lesions in canine arteriosclerosis." *Archives of Pathology and Laboratory Medicine.* 51:288, 1951.

Blankenhorn, D. H., Nessim, S. A., Johnson, R. L., et al. "Beneficial effects of combined colestipol-niacin therapy on coronary atherosclerosis and coronary venous bypass grafts." *Journal of the American Medical Association.* 257(23):3233–40, June 19, 1987.

Blondal, T. "Controlled trial of nicotine polacrilex gum with supportive measures." *Archives of Internal Medicine.* 149(8):1818–21, August 1989.

Bohlin, G., Eliasson, K., Hjemdahl, P., et al. "Pace variation and control of work pace as related to cardiovascular, neuroendocrine, and subjective responses." *Biological Psychology.* 23(3):247–63, December 1986.

Bourassa, M., et al. "Progression of obstructive coronary artery disease 5 to 7 years after aortocoronary bypass surgery." *Circulation.* 58(Suppl 1): I100, January–December 1978.

Brown, G., Albers, J. J., Fisher, L. D., et al. "Regression of coronary artery disease as a result of intensive lipid-lowering therapy in men with high levels of apolipoprotein B." *New England Journal of Medicine.* 323(19):1289–98, November 8, 1990.

Brunner, D., Manelis, G., Modan, M., et al. "Physical activity at work and the incidence of myocardial infarction, angina pectoris and death due to ischemic heart disease. An epidemiological study in Israeli collective settlements (Kibbutzim)." *Journal of Chronic Diseases.* 27(4):217–33, July 1974.

Bruschke, A. V., Wijers, T. S., Kolsters, W., Landmann, J. "The anatomic evolution of coronary artery disease demonstrated by coronary arteriography in 256 nonoperated patients." *Circulation.* 63(3):527–36, March 1981.

Buchwald, H., Varco, R. L., Matts, J. P., et al. "Effect of partial ileal bypass surgery on mortality and morbidity from coronary heart disease in patients with hypercholesterolemia." *New England Journal of Medicine.* 323(14):946–55, October 4, 1990.

Buell, P., Breslow, L. "Mortality from coronary heart disease in California men who work long hours." *Journal of Chronic Diseases.* 11(6):615, June 1960.

Buja, L. M., Kita, T., Goldstein, J. L., Watanabe, Y., Brown, M. S. "Cellular pathology of progressive atherosclerosis in the W.H.H.L. rabbit. An animal model of familial hypercholesterolemia." *Arteriosclerosis.* 3(1):87–101, January–February 1983.

Bulkley, B. H., Hutchins, G. M. "Accelerated 'atherosclerosis.' A morphologic study of 97 saphenous vein coronary artery bypass grafts." *Circulation.* 55(1):163–69, January 1977.

Cairns, J. A., Gent, M., Singer, J., et al. "Aspirin, sulfinpyrazone, or both in unstable angina. Results of a Canadian multi-center trial." *New England Journal of Medicine.* 313(22):1369–75, November 28, 1985.

Campeau, L., Enjalbert, M., Lesperance, J., et al. "Atherosclerosis and late closure of aortocoronary saphenous vein grafts: Sequential angiographic studies at 2 weeks, 1 year, 5 to 7 years, and 10 to 12 years after surgery." *Circulation.* 68(3 Pt 2):II1–7, September 1983.

———. "The relation of risk factors to the development of atherosclerosis in saphenous-vein bypass grafts and the progression of disease in the native circulation." *New England Journal of Medicine.* 311(21):1329–32, November 22, 1984.

Carew, T. E., Schwenke, D., Steinberg, D. "Antiatherogenic effect of probucol unrelated to its hypercholesterolemic effect: Evidence that antioxidants in vivo can selectively inhibit low density lipoprotein degradation in macrophage-rich fatty streaks and slow the progression of atherosclerosis in the Watanabe heritable hyperlipidemic rabbit." *Proceedings of the National Academy of Sciences of the United States of America.* 84(21):7725–29, November 1987.

Carlson, L. A., Bottiger, L. E. "Risk factors for ischemic heart disease in men and women. Results of a 19-year follow-up of the Stockholm perspective study." *Acta Medica Scandinavica.* 218, 207, 1985.

Carrington, P. *Freedom in Meditation.* Garden City, NY: Doubleday, 1977.

Chesebro, J. H., Fuster, V., Elveback, L. R., et al. "Effect of dipyridamole and aspirin on late vein-graft patency after coronary bypass operations." *New England Journal of Medicine.* 310(4):209–14, January 26, 1984.

Clynes, M. Toward a View of Man. In M. Clynes and J. H. Milsum, *Biomedical Engineering Systems.* New York: McGraw-Hill, 1970.

Coronary Artery Surgery Study (CASS). "A randomized trial of coronary artery bypass surgery. Survival Data." *Circulation.* 68(5):939–50, November 1983.

Daoud, A. S., et al. "Regression of advanced atherosclerosis in swine." *Archives of Pathology and Laboratory Medicine.* 100(7):372–79, July 1976.

Davis, M., McKay, M., Isshelan, E. R. *The Relaxation and Stress Reduction Workbook.* 2nd ed. Oakland, CA: New Harbinger Publishers, 1982.

DePace, N. L., Dowinsky, S. K. Prevention of Further Atherosclerosis in Coronary Artery Bypass Graft Patients. In M. N. Kotler and A. Alfieri, eds., *Cardiac and Non-Cardiac Complications of Open Heart Surgery: Prevention, Diagnosis and Treatment.* Mount Kisco, NY: Futura Publishing Company, 1992.

DePalma, R. G., Klein, L., Bellon, E. M., Koletsky, S. "Regression of atherosclerotic plaques in rhesus monkeys. Angiographic, morphologic, and angiochemical changes." *Archives of Surgery.* 115(11):1268–78, November 1980.

Dishman, R. K. "Medical psychology in exercise and sport." *Medical Clinics of North America.* 69(1):123–43, January 1985.

Eliot, R. S., ed. *Stress and the Heart.* Mount Kisco, NY: Futura Publishing Company, 1988.

Favaloro, R. G., Effler, D. B., Groves, L. K., et al. "Severe segmental obstruction of the left main coronary artery and its divisions. Surgical treatment by the saphenous vein graft technique." *Journal of Thoracic and Cardiovascular Surgery.* 60(4):469–82, October 1970.

Folsom, A. R., Caspersen, C. J., Taylor, H. L., et al. "Leisure time physical activity and its relationship to coronary risk factors in a population-based sample." The Minnesota Heart Survey. *American Journal of Epidemiology.* 121(4):570–79, April 1985.

Forem, J. *Transcendental Meditator.* New York: Dutton, 1974.

Frankenhaeuser, M. "Behavior and circulating catecholamines." *Brain Research.* 31(2):241–62, August 1971.

————. Experimental Approaches to the Study of Human Behavior as Related to Neuroendocrine Functions. In L. Levi, ed., *Society, Stress and Disease.* Oxford: Oxford University Press, 1971.

————, Johansson, G. "Task demand as reflected in catecholamine excretion and heart rate." *Journal of Human Stress.* 2(1):15–23, March 1976.

————, Rissler, A. "Catecholamine output during relaxation and anticipation." *Perceptual and Motor Skills.* 30(3):745–46, June 1970.

Franks, P., Harp, J., Bell, B. "Randomized, controlled trial of clonidine for smoking cessation in a primary care setting." *Journal of the American Medical Association.* 262(21):3011–13, December 1989.

Frick, M. H., Elo, O., Haapa, K., et al. "Helsinki Heart Study: Primary-prevention trial with gemfibrozil in middle-aged men with dyslipidemia. Safety of treatment, changes in risk factors, and incidence of coronary heart disease." *New England Journal of Medicine.* 317(20):1237–45, November 12, 1987.

Friedman, M., et al. "Alteration of Type A behavior and its effect on cardiac recurrences in post-myocardial infarction patients: Summary results of the Recurrent Coronary Prevention Project." *American Heart Journal.* 112(4):653–65, October 1986.

————, Byers, S. O. "Observations concerning the evolution of atherosclerosis in the rabbit after cessation of cholesterol feeding." *American Journal of Pathology.* 43:349–59, September 1963.

————, Rosenman, R. H. "Association of a specific overt behavior pattern with blood and cardiovascular findings: Blood cholesterol level, blood clotting time, incidence of arcus senilis, and clinical coronary artery disease." *Journal of the American Medical Association.* 169:1286, March 1959.

Froelicher, V., Jensen, D., Sullivan, M. "A randomized trial of the effects of exercise training after coronary artery bypass surgery." *Archives of Internal Medicine.* 145(4):689–92, April 1985.

Fuster, V., Badimon, L., Cohen, M., et al. "Insights into the pathogenesis of acute ischemic syndromes." *Circulation.* 77(6):1213–20, June 1988.

Glassman, A. H., Stetner, F., Walsh, B. T., et al. "Heavy smokers, smoking cessation and clonidine." *Journal of the American Medical Association.* 259(19):2863–66, May 1988.

Goldman, S., Copeland, J., Moritz, T., et al. "Effect of antiplatelet therapy on late graft patency after coronary artery bypass grafting." VA Cooperative Study No. 207. Abstract 37, Annual Scientific Session, American College of Cardiology. *Journal of the American College of Cardiology.* II(No. 2, Suppl A):152A, 1988.

Gordon, B., Chang, S., Kavanagh, M., et al. "The effects of lipid lowering on diabetic retinopathy." *American Journal of Ophthalmology.* 112(4):385–91, October 1991.

Gown, A. M., Tsukada, T., Ross, R. "Human atherosclerosis. II. Immunocytochemical analysis of the cellular composition of human atherosclerotic lesions." *American Journal of Pathology.* 125(1):191–207, October 1986.

Green, G. E., Stertzer, S. H., Gordon, R. B., et al. "Anastomosis of the internal mammary artery to the distal left anterior descending coronary artery." *Circulation.* 41(Suppl 5):II79–85, May 1970.

Grondin, C. M., Campeau, L., Lesperance, J., et al. "Comparison of late changes in internal mammary artery and saphenous vein grafts in two consecutive series of patients 10 years after operation." *Circulation.* 70(3 Pt 2):208–12, September 1984.

Guthaner, D. F., Robert, E. W., Alderman, E. L., Wexler, L. "Long-term

serial angiographic studies after coronary artery bypass surgery."
Circulation. 60(2):250–59, August 1979.

Hartung, G. H., Rangel, R. "Exercise training in post-myocardial infarction patients: Comparison of results with high risk coronary and post-bypass patients." *Archives of Physical Medicine and Rehabilitation.* 62(4):147–50, April 1981.

Hecker, M., Chesney, M. A., Black, G. W., et al. "Coronary-prone behaviors in the Western Collaborative Group Study." *Psychosomatic Medicine.* 50:153–64, 1988.

Henry, J. P. Coronary Heart Disease and Arousal of the Adrenal Cortical Axis. In T. M. Dembroski, T. H. Schmidt, and G. Blumchen, eds., *Biobehavioral Bases of Coronary Heart Disease.* New York: S. Karger, 1983.

Hittleman, R. *Introduction to Yoga.* New York: Bantam Books, 1969.

Holmes, T., Rahe, R. "The Social Readjustment Rating Scale." *Journal of Psychosomatic Research.* 11(2):213–18, August 1967.

Hurst, J. W., Whalen, R. E. The Surgical Treatment of Atherosclerotic Coronary Heart Disease. In J. W. Hurst and R. C. Schlant, eds., *The Heart.* Vol. I. *Arteries and Veins.* 7th ed. New York: McGraw-Hill, 1990.

Jarvis, M. J., Hajek, P., Russell, M. A., West, R. J., et al. "Nasal nicotine solution as an aid to cigarette withdrawal: A pilot clinical trial." *British Journal of Addiction.* 82(9):983–88, September 1987.

Johansson, G., Frankenhaeuser, M. "Temporal factors in sympathoadrenomedullary activity following acute behavioral activation." *Biological Psychology.* 1(1):63–73, 1973.

Johnson, J. V. *The Impact of Workplace Social Support Job Demands and Work Control upon Cardiovascular Disease in Sweden.* Department of Psychology, Report No 1. Stockholm: University of Stockholm, 1986.

Johnson, W. D., Flemma, R. J., Lepley, D. Jr., et al. "Extended treatment of severe coronary artery disease: A total surgical approach." *Annals of Surgery.* 170(3):460–70, September 1969.

Kane, J. P., Malloy, M. J., Ports, T. A., et al. "Regression of coronary atherosclerosis during treatment of familial hypercholesterolemia with combined drug regimens." *Journal of the American Medical Association.* 264:3007–12, 1990.

Kannel, W. B., Dawber, T., et al. "Factors of risk in the development of coronary heart disease—six-year follow-up experience. The Framingham Study." *Annals of Internal Medicine.* 55(1):33–48, July 1961.

———, Neaton, J. D., Wentworth, D., et al. "Overall and coronary heart disease mortality rates in relation to major risk factors in 325,348 men screened for the MRFIT." Multiple Risk Factor Intervention Trial. *American Heart Journal.* 112(4):825–36, October 1986.

———, Sorlie P. "Some health benefits of physical activity: The Framingham Study." *Archives of Internal Medicine.* 139(8):857–61, August 1979.

Karasek, R., Baker, D., Marxer, F., et al. "Job decision latitude, job demands, and cardiovascular diseases: A prospective study of Swedish men." *American Journal of Public Health.* 71(7):694–705, July 1981.

———, Triantis, K., Chaudhry, S. "Coworker and supervisor support as moderators of associations between task characteristics and mental strain." *Journal of Occupational Behavior.* 3:181, 1982.

Keys, A., ed. "Coronary heart disease in seven countries." *Circulation.* 41(Suppl 1):I1–I211, April 1970.

Kita, T., Nagano, Y., Yokode, M., et al. "Probucol prevents the progression of atherosclerosis in Watanabe heritable hyperlipidemic rabbit: An animal model for familial hypercholesterolemia." *Proceedings of the National Academy of Sciences of the United States of America.* 84(16):5928–31, August 1987.

Klein, L. W., Pichard, A. D., Holt, J., et al. "Effects of chronic tobacco smoking on the coronary circulation." *Journal of the American College of Cardiology.* 1(2 Pt 1):421–26, February 1983.

Kramer, J. R., Matsuda, Y., Mulligan, J.C., et al. "Progression of coronary atherosclerosis." *Circulation.* 63(3):519–26, March 1981.

Kromhout, D., et al. "The inverse relation between fish consumption and 20-year mortality from coronary heart disease." *New England Journal of Medicine.* 312(19):1205–09, May 9, 1985.

LaCroix, A., Haynes, S. Gender Differences in the Health Effects of Workplace Roles. In R. C. Barnett, L. Biener, and G. Baruch, eds., *Gender and Stress.* New York: Free Press, 1987.

Leaf, A., Weber, P. C. "Cardiovascular effects of n-3 fatty acids." *New England Journal of Medicine.* 318(9):549–57, March 3, 1988.

LeCron, L. *Self-Hypnotism.* New York: New American Library, 1970.

Leon, A. S., Connett, J., Jacobs, D. R., Jr., et al. "Leisure-time physical activity levels and risk of coronary heart disease and death: The Multiple Risk Factor Intervention Trial." *Journal of the American Medical Association.* 258(17):2388–95, November 6, 1987.

LeShan, L. *How to Meditate.* New York: Bantam Books, 1974.

Levy, R. I., Brensike, J. F., Epstein, S. E., et al. "The influence of changes in lipid values induced by cholestyramine and diet on progression of coronary artery disease: Results of NHLBI Type II Coronary Intervention Study." *Circulation.* 69(2):325–37, February 1984.

Lewis, H. D., Jr., Davis, J. W., Archibald, D. G., et al. "Protective effects of aspirin against acute myocardial infarction and death in men with unstable angina. Results of a Veterans Administration Cooperative Study." *New England Journal of Medicine.* 309(7):396–403, August 18, 1983.

Lidell, L. *The Sivananda Companion to Yoga.* New York: Simon & Schuster, 1983.

The Lipid Research Clinics Coronary Primary Prevention Trial Results. I. "Reduction in incidence of coronary heart disease." *Journal of the American Medical Association.* 251(3):351–64, January 1984.

Lundberg, U., Frankenhaeuser, M. "Pituitary-adrenal and sympathetic-adrenal correlates of distress and effort." *Journal of Psychosomatic Research.* 24(3–4):125–30, 1980.

Luthe, W. "Autogenic training: Method, research and application in medicine." *American Journal of Psychotherapy.* 17(2):174–80, April 1963.

Malinow, M. R. "Atherosclerosis: Progression, regression, and resolution." *American Heart Journal.* 108(6):1523–37, December 1984.

Manuck, S. B., Kaplan, J. R., Matthews, K. A. "Behavioral antecedents of coronary heart disease and atherosclerosis." *Arteriosclerosis.* 6(1):2–14, January–February 1986.

Markowe, H. L., Marmot, M. G., Shipley, M. J., et al. "Fibrinogen: A possible link between social class and coronary heart disease."

British Medical Journal—Clinical Research. 291(6505):1312–14, November 9, 1985.

Matarazzo, M., DePace, N. L. "Hepatotoxicity with long-term treatment of hyperlipidemia with niacin and lovastatin." *Clinical Research.* 40(2):272A, 1992.

McMeans, J. W. "Superficial fatty streaks of arteries: An experimental study." *Journal of Medical Research.* 34:41, 1916.

Morris, J. N., Chave, S. P., Adam, C., et al. "Vigorous exercise in leisure-time and the incidence of coronary heart disease." *The Lancet.* 1(799):333–39, February 1973.

Mudge, G. H., Jr., et al. "Reflex increase in coronary vascular resistance in patients with ischemic heart disease." *New England Journal of Medicine.* 295(24):1333–37, December 1976.

Multiple Risk Factor Intervention Trial Research Group. "Mortality rates after 10.5 years for participants in the Multiple Risk Factor Intervention Trial." *Journal of the American Medical Association.* 263(13):1795–801, April 1990.

———. Multiple Risk Factor Intervention Trial: "Risk factor changes and mortality results." *Journal of the American Medical Association.* 248(12):1465–77, September 1982.

Nagai, Y., Nakamura, T., Takemura, K., et al. "Effect of combined treatment with pravastatin, probucol and cholestyramine for cholesterol reduction and xanthoma regression in patients with familial hypercholesterolemia." *Arteriosclerosis.* Abstract. 9(5):754a, September–October 1989.

Nararjo, C., Ornstein, R. *The Psychology of Meditation.* New York: Viking Press, 1971.

Ornish, D., Brown, S. E., Scherwitz, L. W., et al. "Can lifestyle changes reverse coronary heart disease?" *The Lancet.* 336(8708):129–33, July 21, 1990.

Ornish, S. A., Zisook, S., McAdams, L. A. "Effects of transdermal clonidine treatment on withdrawal symptoms associated with smoking cessation." *Archives of Internal Medicine.* 148(9):2027–31, September 1988.

Paffenbarger, R. S., Gima. A. S., Laughlin. E., et al. "Characteristics of longshoremen-related fatal coronary heart disease and stroke." *American Journal of Public Health.* 61(7):1362–70, July 1971.

Paffenbarger, R. S., Jr., Hyde, R. T., Wing, A. L., et al. "Physical activity, all-cause mortality, and longevity of college alumni." *New England Journal of Medicine.* 314(10):605–13, March 6, 1986.

Palac, R. T., Hwang, M. H., Meadows, W. R., et al. "Progression of coronary artery disease in medically and surgically treated patients 5 years after randomization." *Circulation.* 64(2 Pt 2):II17–21, August 1981.

Physicians' Health Study Research Group. "Preliminary Report: Findings from the aspirin component of the ongoing Physicians' Health Study." *New England Journal of Medicine.* 318(4):262–64, January 1988.

The Pooling Project Research Group. "Relationship of blood pressure, serum cholesterol, smoking habit, relative weight and ECG abnormalities to incidence of major coronary events: Final report of the Pooling Project." *Journal of Chronic Diseases.* 31(4):201–306, April 1978.

Ragland, D. R., Brand, R. J. "Type A behavior and mortality from coronary heart disease." *New England Journal of Medicine.* 318(2):65–69, January 14, 1988.

[Anonymous.] "Randomized trial of intravenous streptokinase, oral aspirin, both, or neither among 17,187 cases of suspected acute myocardial infarction: ISIS-2." ISIS-2 (Second International Study of Infarct Survival) Collaborative Group. *The Lancet.* 2(8607):349–60, August 1988.

Ravi, Subbiah M. T., Dicke, B. A., Kottke, B. A., et al. "Regression of naturally occurring atherosclerotic lesions in pigeon aorta by intestinal bypass surgery." *Atherosclerosis.* 31(2):117–24, October 1978.

Report from the Committee of Principal Investigators. "A cooperative trial in the primary prevention of ischemic heart disease using clofibrate." *British Heart Journal.* 40:1069–1118, October 1978.

Report of the National Cholesterol Education Program Expert Panel. "Detection, evaluation and treatment of high blood cholesterol in adults." *Archives of Internal Medicine.* 148(1):36–69, January 1988.

Rose, J. E., et al. "Transdermal nicotine facilitates smoking cessation." *Clinical Pharmacology and Therapeutics.* 47(3):323–30, March 1990.

Roth, G. J., Majerus, P. W. "The mechanism of the effect of aspirin on human platelets. I. Acetylation of a particular fraction protein." *Journal of Clinical Investigation.* 56(3):624–32, September 1975.

Rozanski, A., Bairey, C. N., Krantz, D. S., et al. "Mental stress and the induction of silent myocardial ischemia in patients with coronary artery disease." *New England Journal of Medicine.* 318(16):1005–12, April 21, 1988.

Russek, H. L., Zohman, B. L. "Relative significance of heredity, diet and occupational stress in coronary heart disease of young adults." *American Journal of Science.* 235:266, 1958.

Schwartz, M. S. *Biofeedback, The Practitioner's Guide.* New York: Guilford Press, 1987.

[Anonymous.] "Secondary prevention of vascular disease by prolonged antiplatelet treatment." Antiplatelet Trialists' Collaboration. *British Medical Journal—Clinical Research.* 296(6618):320–31, January 1988.

Shekelle, R. B., Hulley, S. B., Neaton, J. D., et al. "The MRFIT behavior pattern study. II. Type A behavior and incidence of coronary heart disease." *American Journal of Epidemiology.* 122(4):559–70, October 1985.

Shepherd, J. T., Vanhoutte, P. M. "Spasm of the coronary arteries: Causes and consequences (the scientist's viewpoint)." *Mayo Clinic Proceedings.* 60(1):33–46, January 1985.

Shiomi, M., Ito, T., Watanabe, Y., et al. "Suppression of established atherosclerosis and xanthomas in mature WHHL rabbits by keeping their serum cholesterol levels extremely low." *Atherosclerosis.* 83(1):69–80, July 1990.

Shub, C., Vlietstra, R. E., Smith, H. C., et al. "The unpredictable progression of symptomatic coronary artery disease: A serial clinical-angiographic analysis." *Mayo Clinic Proceedings.* 56(3):155–60, March 1981.

Slattery, M. L., Jacobs, D. R., Jr., Nichaman, M. Z. "Leisure time physical activity and coronary heart disease death. The U.S. Railroad Study." *Circulation.* 79(2):304–11, February 1989.

Small, D. M., et al. "Physicochemical and histological changes in the arterial wall of nonhuman primates during progression and regression of atherosclerosis." *Journal of Clinical Investigation.* 73(6):1590–1605, June 1984.

Stevens, R., Hanson, P. "Comparison of supervised and unsupervised exercise training after coronary bypass surgery." *American Journal of Cardiology.* 53(11):1524–28, June 1, 1984.

Stokes, J., III. Dyslipidemia as a Risk Factor for Cardiovascular Disease and Untimely Death: The Framingham Study. In J. Stokes III and M. Mancini, eds., *Dyslipidemia: The Most Powerful Modifiable Risk Factor. Atherosclerosis Reviews.* New York: Raven Press Ltd., 1988.

————, Rigotti, N. A. "The health consequences of cigarette smoking and the internist's role in smoking cessation." *Advances in Internal Medicine.* 33:431–60, 1988.

Tappan, F. M. *Healing Massage Techniques: Holistic, Classic, and Emerging.* Norwalk, CN: Appleton & Lange, 1988.

Taylor, H. L., Blackburn, H., Brozek, J., et al. "Railroad employees in the United States." *Acta Medica Scandinavica.* 460(suppl):55, 1967.

Tofler, G. H., et al. "Analysis of possible triggers of acute myocardial infarction (The MILIS Study)." *American Journal of Cardiology.* 66(1):22–27, July 1, 1990.

van Dijkhuizen, N., Reiche, H. "Psychosocial stress in industry: A heartache for middle management?" *Psychotherapy and Psychosomatics.* 34(2–3):124–34, 1980.

Wallace, R. K. "Physiological effects of transcendental meditation." *Science.* 167(926):1751–54, March 1970.

Ward, M. M., Mefford, I. N., Parker, S. D., et al. "Epinephrine and norepinephrine responses in continuously collected human plasma to a series of stressors." *Psychosomatic Medicine.* 45(6):471–86, December 1983.

Weber, G., et al. "Regression of arteriosclerotic lesions in rhesus monkey aortas after regression diet. Scanning and transmission electron microscope observations of the endothelium." *Atherosclerosis.* 26(4):535–47, April 1977.

Wilens, S. L. "The resorption of arterial atheromatous deposits in wasting disease." *American Journal of Pathology.* 25:793, 1947.

Wilson, P. W., Garrison, R. J., Abbott, R. D., Castelli, W. P. "Factors associated with lipoprotein cholesterol levels: The Framingham Study." *Arteriosclerosis.* 3(3):273–81, May–June 1983.

Wissler, R. W., Vesselinovitch, D. "Combined effects of cholestyramine and probucol on regression of atherosclerosis in rhesus monkey aortas." *Applied Pathology.* 1(2):89–96, 1983.

Yamamoto, A., Matsuzawa, Y., Yokoyama, S., et al. "Effects of probucol on xanthomata regression in familial hypercholesterolemia."
American Journal of Cardiology. 57(16):29H–35H, June 27,
1986.

Index